CONCISE GUIDE TO
Evaluation and Management of Sleep Disorders

American Psychiatric Press
CONCISE GUIDES

Robert E. Hales, M.D.
Series Editor

CONCISE GUIDE TO

Evaluation and Management of Sleep Disorders

Martin Reite, M.D., A.C.P.
Director and Professor of Psychiatry

Kim Nagel, M.D.
Associate Director and Assistant Clinical Professor of Psychiatry

John Ruddy, M.D., A.C.P.
Associate Director and Assistant Clinical Professor of Psychiatry

Sleep Disorders Center
Department of Psychiatry
University of Colorado Health Sciences Center
Denver, Colorado 80204

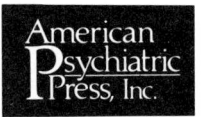

1400 K Street, N.W.
Washington, DC 20005

Copyright © 1990 American Psychiatric Press, Inc.
ALL RIGHTS RESERVED
Manufactured in the United States of America

First Edition 93 92 91 90 4 3 2 1
The paper used in this publication meets the minimum requirements of the American National Standard for Information Sciences—Permanence of Paper for Printed Library Materials, ANSI Z39.48—1984. ∞

Library of Congress Cataloging-in-Publication Data

Reite, Martin.
  Concise guide to evaluation and management of sleep disorders / Martin Reite, Kim Nagel, John Ruddy.—1st ed.
    p. cm.—(Concise guides / American Psychiatric Press)
  Includes bibliographical references.
  ISBN 0-88048-334-2 (alk. paper)
    1. Sleep disorders. I. Nagel, Kim, 1953– . II. Ruddy, John, 1954– . III. Title. IV. Series: Concise guides (American Psychiatric Press)
    [DNLM: 1. Sleep Disorders—diagnosis. 2. Sleep Disorders—therapy. WM 188 R379c]
  RC547.R45 1990
  616.8'498—dc20
  DNLM/DLC
  for Library of Congress   89-17711
                                                 CIP

Note: The authors have worked to ensure that all information in this book concerning drug dosages, schedules, and routes of administration is accurate as of the time of publication and consistent with standards set by the U.S. Food and Drug Administration and the general medical community. As medical research and practice advance, however, therapeutic standards may change. For this reason and because human and mechanical errors sometimes occur, we recommend that readers follow the advice of a physician who is directly involved in their care or the care of a member of their family.

Because the use of L-tryptophan has recently (Fall 1989) been implicated in an increased incidence of eosinophilia, the authors advise against the prescribing and use of this agent, as discussed in this book, until the issue is resolved.

The opinions or assertions contained herein are the private ones of Dr. Hales and are not to be construed as official or reflecting the views of the Department of Defense, Letterman Army Medical Center, or the Department of the Army. This book was prepared in the Series Editor's private capacity. Neither government-financed time nor supplies were used in connection with this project.

Books published by the American Psychiatric Press, Inc., represent the views and opinions of the individual authors and do not necessarily represent the policies and opinions of the Press or the American Psychiatric Association.

CONTENTS

Introduction to Concise Guides	ix
Acknowledgments	xiii

1. OVERVIEW OF SLEEP DISORDERS MEDICINE ... 1
- Symptom Approach to Sleep Disorders ... 2
- Sleep Disorders Centers ... 8
- References ... 13
- Additional Reading ... 13

2. SLEEP PHYSIOLOGY AND PATHOLOGY ... 14
- Sleep Architecture ... 14
- Ontogeny of Sleep Architecture and Sleep Patterns ... 19
- Physiology and Neurophysiology of Sleep ... 20
- References ... 26
- Additional Readings ... 27

3. TRANSIENT AND CHRONIC INSOMNIAS ... 27
- Transient Insomnias ... 27
- Evaluation of Chronic Insomnia ... 28
- Insomnia Secondary to Substance Abuse and Drug Dependency ... 33
- Circadian Rhythm-Based Sleep Disorders ... 40
- Periodic Limb Movements (Nocturnal Myoclonus) and Restless Leg Syndrome ... 51
- Sleep Apnea Insomnia ... 59
- Psychophysiological Insomnia ... 62
- Rare Causes of Insomnia ... 72
- References ... 74
- Additional Readings ... 76

4. EXCESSIVE SLEEPINESS DISORDERS ... 76
- Evaluation of Excessive Daytime Sleepiness ... 76
- Narcolepsy ... 80
- Hypersomnia Due to Sleep-Related Breathing Disorders ... 89
- Other Causes of Excessive Daytime Sleepiness ... 101

    References.................................... 106
    Additional Readings 107

5. PARASOMNIAS................................. 108
    Parasomnias Associated With REM Sleep........... 108
    Sleepwalking and Night Terrors 111
    Other Parasomnias 117
    References.................................... 121

6. MEDICAL AND PSYCHIATRIC DISORDERS AND SLEEP................................. 122
    Medical Disorders and Sleep 122
    Psychiatric Disorders and Sleep 127
    References.................................... 141
    Additional Reading 142

7. USE OF SEDATIVE-HYPNOTIC AGENTS 142
    Choice of a Hypnotic Agent 143
    Longer-Term Use of Sedative-Hypnotic Agents....... 151
    References.................................... 152
    Additional Readings 152

8. SPECIAL PROBLEMS AND POPULATIONS 152
    Sleep Problems in Children 152
    Enuresis...................................... 159
    Sleep in the Elderly............................ 163
    Sleep Problems During Pregnancy 169
    Insomnia without Objective Findings.............. 174
    References.................................... 175

Index 177

INTRODUCTION

to the *American Psychiatric Press Concise Guides*

The *American Psychiatric Press Concise Guides* series provides, in a most accessible format, practical information for psychiatrists—and especially for psychiatry residents and medical students—working in such varied treatment settings as inpatient psychiatry services, outpatient clinics, consultation/liaison services, and private practice. The *Concise Guides* are meant to complement the more detailed information to be found in lengthier psychiatry texts.

The *Concise Guides* address topics of greatest concern to psychiatrists in clinical practice. The books in this series contain a detailed table of contents, along with an index, tables, and charts, for easy access; and their size, designed to fit into a lab coat pocket, makes them a convenient source of information. The number of references has been limited to those most relevant to the material presented.

The authors of this *Concise Guide* are all involved in the diagnosis and treatment of patients with sleep disorders. Dr. Martin Reite, Professor of Psychiatry at the University of Colorado School of Medicine, is Director of the University Sleep Disorders Center. Drs. Kim Nagel and John Ruddy are his two Associate Directors; they both are also Assistant Clinical Professors of Psychiatry in the Department of Psychiatry at the University of Colorado. Dr. Reite has had an outstanding academic career, having published over 100 scientific articles, books, and book chapters. He serves on several journal editorial boards and has been very active in developing neurobiological research projects at the University of Colorado. These three authors have teamed up to produce an excellent, concise overview of the fascinating area of sleep and sleep disorders.

As implied in the title, Drs. Reite, Nagel, and Ruddy have emphasized the evaluation and management of sleep disorders. They begin the book by discussing classification issues, with a focus upon a symptom approach to the recognition of sleep problems. The authors also outline how common sleep disorders are and how they often may be ignored or missed not only by psychiatrists but also by physicians in other specialties. The reader is then provided with basic information necessary to understand sleep: sleep architecture, sleep patterns, and the physiology and neurophysiology of sleep. With this sound scientific background, the authors then turn their attention to a systematic discussion of three major categories of sleep disorders: transient and chronic insomnias, excessive sleepiness disorders, and parasomnias.

Within the overall categories of transient and chronic insomnias, the authors focus their discussion upon the following specific disorders: insomnia secondary to substance abuse and drug dependency, circadian rhythm-based sleep disorders, nocturnal myoclonus and restless leg syndrome, sleep apnea insomnia, psychophysiological insomnia, and other rare causes of insomnia. In their chapter on transient and chronic insomnias, they emphasize the value of a symptomatic evaluation of chronic insomnia to rule out medical causes and other treatable conditions. The authors then turn their attention to excessive sleepiness disorders: narcolepsy and hypersomnia due to sleep-related breathing disorders. Finally, they discuss the parasomnias, with an emphasis upon those parasomnias associated with REM sleep and those associated with Stage 3 and Stage 4 sleep (e.g., sleep walking and night terrors).

In other chapters, Drs. Reite, Nagel, and Ruddy discuss the importance of recognizing how medical and psychiatric disorders may affect sleep and how physicians should select a sedative-hypnotic agent, if necessary, to treat a sleep disorder. They discuss issues concerning the use of both benzodiazepine and nonbenzodiazepine hypnotic agents, as well as problems associated with longer-term use of these drugs. The authors conclude their book by discussing three special populations who frequently have sleep problems: children, the elderly, and pregnant women. With regard to children, they emphasize an approach to treating enuresis in this population.

This is a marvelous book that includes a wealth of information. Dr. Reite and his colleagues have included many outstanding figures to explain information in the text, as well as equally excellent tables. Readers should be pleased with the clear and precise prose and the book's clinical relevance. The material contained in this book is new and is of the highest quality. The authors have included a number of recent references and have made a thorough and careful review of the literature. They address many controversies in the sleep field and provide a sound basis for their treatment recommendations.

The **Concise Guide to Evaluation and Management of Sleep Disorders** is a beautifully written, pocket-sized book that should be of invaluable assistance to psychiatrists and other mental health professionals. In particular, residents and medical students should find it an excellent addition to their practical medical library.

Robert E. Hales, M.D.
Series Editor
American Psychiatric Press Concise Guides

Concise Guide Series Titles

Clinical Psychiatry
Steven L. Dubovsky, MD

Clinical Psychiatry and the Law
Robert I. Simon, MD

Consultation Psychiatry
Michael G. Wise, MD, and James R. Rundell, MD

Somatic Therapies in Psychiatry
Laurence B. Guttmacher, MD

Group Psychotherapy
Sophia Vinogradov, MD, and Irvin D. Yalom, MD

Assessment and Management of Violent Patients
Kenneth Tardiff, MD, MPH

Treatment of Alcoholism and Addictions
Richard J. Frances, MD, and John E. Franklin, MD

Laboratory and Diagnostic Testing in Psychiatry
Richard B. Rosse, MD; Alexis A. Giese, MD; Stephen I. Deutsch, MD; and John M. Morihisa, MD

Evaluation and Management of Sleep Disorders
Martin L. Reite, MD; Kim E. Nagel, MD; and John R. Ruddy, MD

Geriatric Psychiatry
Edward Spar, MD, and Asenath LaRue, MD

ACKNOWLEDGMENTS

This work was completed while M. Reite was a Fellow at the Center for Advanced Study in the Behavioral Sciences, Stanford, California. Grateful acknowledgment is made for financial support provided by the John D. and Catherine T. MacArthur Foundation, and by U.S. Public Health Service Research Scientist Award No. MH-46335. Special thanks are extended to Katherine Holm, Deanna Knickerbocker, Virginia Heaton, and the staff at the Center for Advanced Study, and to Lisa Higgs, Linda Greco-Sanders, and Sheryl Juarez at the University of Colorado Health Sciences Center, for their expert assistance in the preparation of this manuscript.

OVERVIEW OF SLEEP DISORDERS MEDICINE

Sleep complaints are among the most common voiced by our patients. Not sleeping enough or sleeping too much, trouble falling or staying asleep, not feeling rested during the day, or peculiar, unusual, or annoying things occurring during sleep may affect almost everyone at one time or another. It has been estimated that over 20% of the adult population experience one or more bouts of chronic insomnia at some time during their lives (1). Sleep-related breathing disorders are increasingly recognized as a major cause of morbidity, if not mortality. Most physicians and other clinicians have not yet had the opportunity to learn a great deal about the relatively new area of sleep disorders medicine, and thus they may not be able to offer their patients the latest in diagnosis and management. Indeed, not too long ago, complaints of insomnia were handled with a routine barbiturate prescription, and complaints of excessive daytime sleepiness (EDS) were handled by a psychiatric referral. We simply did not know what else to do; the fact that most sleep complaints have specific separable causes and treatments was until recently unknown. Even now, education in sleep disorders medicine is still marginal at best in many if not most clinical training programs.

This volume is designed to provide the practicing clinician with (a) a practical approach to the differential diagnosis and effective treatment of patients with sleep complaints and disorders, and (b) a succinct, up-to-date summary of sleep disorders medicine. We emphasize a conceptual framework to facilitate the differential diagnosis, and decision trees to facilitate such evaluation. Because it is difficult to be comprehensive or thorough in this rapidly expanding field, references and suggestions for additional reading are given at the end of each chapter, citing recent articles and books that provide in-depth coverage for those interested. Our goal is to provide a useful entré to this new area, with sufficient detail to permit the intelligent evaluation and management of most patients, as well as to provide indications as to where to find the necessary information for the more complicated and obscure problems. We hope also to help spark an interest in this important area, and encourage others to become involved as sleep disorders clinicians and researchers.

■ SYMPTOM APPROACH TO SLEEP DISORDERS

Sleep disorders medicine has not yet reached the point where we can make our diagnoses based upon a thorough understanding of the pathophysiological mechanisms involved, or upon conclusive laboratory studies. We still depend upon the patient to tell us the symptoms, and our diagnostic nomenclatures have been based predominantly upon these symptoms. Typically, patients' complaints will fall into three broad areas: "Doctor, I can't sleep" (i.e., the insomnias); "Doctor, I sleep too much" (i.e., EDS); or "Doctor, strange things happen when I sleep" (i.e., the parasomnias).

DIAGNOSTIC NOMENCLATURES FOR SLEEP DISORDERS

The International Classification of Diseases–Ninth Revision (ICD-9-CM) classifies sleep disorders in three locations—under Mental Disorders (codes 307.40–307.49), under class 347 (narcolepsy), and in the section entitled Symptoms, Signs, and Ill-defined Conditions (codes 780.5–780.59). While generally useful for diagnostic coding, and encompassing most of the common sleep disorders, this organizational approach is not entirely satisfactory.

Perhaps the most widely used current nomenclature for sleep disorders is that developed by the Association of Sleep Disorders Centers (ASDC) (2). This nomenclature is frequently referred to as the DIMS-DOES classification, because it primarily divides sleep disorders based upon whether the complaint is an insomnia (A. DIMS: Disorders of Initiating or Maintaining Sleep) or excessive sleepiness (B. DOES: Disorders of Excessive Somnolence). Circadian rhythm disorders, usually presenting as insomnias, are grouped independently (C. Disorders of the Sleep-Wake Schedule). The unusual things happening during sleep generally fall into the area of the parasomnias (D. Dysfunctions Associated with Sleep, Sleep Stages, or Partial Arousals). This nomenclature attempts to be inclusive of all sleep disorders but suffers from several problems (3), one of which is that being symptom-based, the same pathophysiological entity may show up in more than one place. For example, nocturnal myoclonus, a frequent cause of chronic insomnia, may so disrupt nocturnal sleep as to present as both insomnia (ASDC DIMS Classification A.5.a.) and EDS (ASDC DOES Classification B.5.a.). The ASDC classification is currently in the process of extensive revision by the American Sleep Disorders Association (ASDA) (4). The proposed revision, which should be available by the time the present volume is published, will be entitled the *International Classification of Sleep Disorders* (ICSD). As currently planned, this classification will utilize a multiaxial system for stating and coding diagnosis, to be arranged as follows:

- AXIS A: ICSD classification of Sleep Disorder
- AXIS B: ICD-9-CM classification of procedures and ICSD classification of procedure features
- AXIS C: ICD-9-CM classification of diseases (nonsleep diagnoses)

The classification of sleep disorders will no longer be by symptom, but rather will be broken down as follows:

1. Dyssomnias
   1.A. Endogenous sleep disorders, which are those arising from causes within the body (e.g., psychophysiological insomnia, narcolepsy, obstructive sleep apnea, periodic limb movements [nocturnal myoclonus]).
   1.B. Exogenous sleep disorders, which are those arising from external factors (e.g., drug- and alcohol-induced sleep disorders, high-altitude insomnia, sleep disorders as a result of poor sleep hygiene, and poor limit setting in children).
   1.C. Circadian rhythm sleep disorders (e.g., jet lag, shiftworker sleep disorder, delayed sleep phase syndrome).

2. Parasomnias, or disorders of arousal, partial arousal, and sleep-stage transition.
   - 2.A. Arousal disorders (e.g., sleepwalking, night terrors).
   - 2.B. Sleep-wake transition disorders (e.g., sleeptalking).
   - 2.C. Parasomnias usually associated with rapid eye movement (REM) sleep (e.g., nightmares, sleep paralysis).
   - 2.D. Other parasomnias (e.g., snoring, enuresis).
3. Sleep disorders associated with medical and/or psychiatric disorders.
   - 3.A. Mental disorders.
   - 3.B. Neurological disorders.
   - 3.C. Medical disorders.
4. Proposed sleep disorders, for which there is presently insufficient information to characterize the disorders (e.g., pregnancy-related sleep disorders, short or long sleeper, menstruation-related sleep disorder).

This new classification scheme, which represents a substantial improvement over the one presently in use, begins to address diagnosis based on pathology, a direction made possible by recent advances in our understanding of sleep disorders.

Alternative nomenclatures are also to be found. One such is contained in the DSM-III-R (5). While sleep disorders are not mental disorders (although sleep symptoms may be prominent in some mental disorders, e.g., see Chapter 6), in the past psychiatrists have often been responsible for evaluating patients with sleep complaints. The DSM-III-R nomenclature (Table 1-1) is basically a condensed and limited classification scheme that emphasizes those sleep disorders most likely to be found in a psychiatric practice. It generally does not take advantage of the important diagnostic information often made available by sleep laboratory diagnostic procedures.

THE SYMPTOM APPROACH

The symptom approach, which we use in this book, remains the most useful scheme for the initial evaluation and differential diagnosis of patients with sleep complaints. We must recognize that it does have certain limitations, however. It does not, for

TABLE 1-1. **DSM-III-R classification of sleep disorders**

Dyssomnias

Insomnia disorders
- 307.42 Insomnia related to another mental disorder (nonorganic)
- 780.50 Insomnia related to a known organic factor
- 307.42 Primary insomnia

Hypersomnia disorders
- 307.44 Hypersomnia related to another mental disorder (nonorganic)
- 780.50 Hypersomnia related to a known organic factor
- 780.54 Primary hypersomnia

Sleep-wake schedule disorder
- 307.45 Sleep-wake schedule disorder

Other dyssomnias
- 307.40 Dyssomnias not otherwise specified

Parasomnias

- 307.47 Dream anxiety disorder (nightmare disorder)
- 307.46 Sleep terror disorder
- 307.46 Sleepwalking disorder
- 307.40 Parasomnia not otherwise specified

example, initially separate true disorders of sleep from disorders that affect sleep and so result in similar symptoms. For example, narcolepsy is a true sleep disorder —probably specifically a disorder of REM sleep—that results in a set of symptoms that include EDS. Certain sleep-related breathing disorders (e.g., the obstructive apneas) are not true disorders of sleep; they are really disorders of respiratory-related physiology that nonetheless interfere with sleep and thus result in a set of symptoms that may include EDS. These quite different disorders, from the standpoint of their pathophysiologies, are included in the same broad diagnostic category of DOES, because their presenting symptoms are alike. Similarly, an insomnia caused by a major affective disorder, which may represent a basic disturbance in the regulation of the function and timing of CNS-based sleep systems, and thus may be a true sleep disorder, may be grouped together with a similarly presenting insomnia resulting from sedative-hypnotic abuse or a sleep-related breathing disorder such as central apnea. Again, the pathophysiologies are quite dissimilar, but the disorders are grouped together because of the similar way in which they present and the general similarity of their symptoms.

The symptom approach does facilitate diagnosis, however, after which the diagnostic coding can use other schemes, such as that proposed by the ASDA.

By adopting the symptom approach in this book, we accept the fact that a single pathophysiological entity may show up in more than one place in the classification. We have attempted, however, to cross-reference such occurrences when necessary.

TAKING A SLEEP HISTORY

An accurate history is of paramount importance in our evaluation of sleep disorders. While laboratory studies, such as the polysomnogram (PSG) and the multiple sleep latency test (MSLT), are often very helpful, and often essential, it nonetheless is the history—an accurate assessment of symptoms and their time course, periodicity, and effect on the patient—that is central to making our initial diagnosis or shaping our differential diagnosis. And because sleep laboratory studies are often either too expensive or too inconvenient to obtain on a frequent follow-up basis for the purpose of assessing treatment effectiveness, the patient's ongoing account of his or her symptoms is central to assessing treatment response.

The sleep history involves a careful assessment of the complaint in its medical, environmental, and familial context. The following points should be covered:

- When did the symptoms begin, and what has been their pattern since onset (e.g., Are they persistent, or do they wax and wane in intensity? Are they seasonal?).
- Were there associated medical-, job-, or stress-related factors at the time of onset? Have these factors persisted, and do they relate to intensity of symptoms?
- What makes the symptoms better? What makes them worse? What happens on a vacation?
- What is the impact of the sleep complaint on the patient's life?

- What is the patient's typical daily schedule? Is his or her sleep hygiene adequate (see Chapter 3)?
- Is there a family history of sleep complaints, similar or otherwise?
- What treatments have been prescribed or tried to date, and how effective have they been?
- What drugs has the patient used in the past? What drugs is he or she using at present?

Sources of diagnostic information include the patient, who is usually the one to bring the complaint to us; but other sources might include the bed partner and other family members or friends. It is not infrequent in sleep disorders for someone other than the patient to be the primary complainant, especially when the patient is a child, or when the sleep disorder involves events that occur while the patient is asleep, and of which the patient has no memory. In such cases it is usually quite important to try and obtain such information from another person—either a bed partner in the case of adult patients, or a parent in the case of a child patient. These observers can provide important information often not known by the patient that can greatly facilitate our diagnostic decision making.

The *sleep diary* or *sleep log* can be a most useful adjunct to the history. A careful recording over a 2-week period of time in bed, including associated subjective sleep patterns (time in bed, time asleep, all awakenings, time of final awakening, time out of bed) and other factors, such as meals, activity patterns, drugs and alcohol consumption, and job-related and social events, can provide evidence of periodicity of complaints, association with other factors, etc., that the patient may not otherwise be aware of.

A completed sleep diary can be used to compute estimates of total sleep time (TST), sleep efficiency (SE), number of awakenings during the night, and related numerical indices that can be used to assess subjective symptomatic improvement. The diary can help relate especially bad nights to particular days of the week, stressful events, etc. Evidence of sleeping in on weekends to recoup sleep lost during the week can be useful in uncovering delayed sleep phase syndromes and other disturbances in the rhythmical control of sleep.

■ SLEEP DISORDERS CENTERS

Sleep Disorders Centers provide the capability for both diagnostic evaluation and, if desired, consultation and management of most sleep-related complaints. The ASDA accredits Sleep Disorders Centers based upon evidence that facilities are adequate, and laboratory and clinical personnel appropriately trained, to perform accurate recordings and assessments of sleep disorders. Laboratories specializing only in the evaluation of sleep-related breathing disorders, but not in the entire range of sleep disorders, can receive separate accreditation as Laboratories for Sleep Related Breathing Disorders.

The ASDA is a private nonprofit organization whose main concern is assuring maintenance of high, and shared, standards in the assessment of sleep disorders. The ASDA additionally supports a program of certification of personnel by examination to assure standards of those individuals supervising Sleep Disorders Centers and interpreting laboratory studies. The M.D. and/or Ph.D. who completes a period of formal training followed by successful passing of a two-part written and oral examination may be certified as an Accredited Clinical Polysomnographer (ACP).

ASDA accreditation for Sleep Disorders Centers entails a formal application procedure and a site visit by an ASDA representative to ensure that all requirements have been complied with. Further information on application procedure can be obtained from the American Sleep Disorders Association, 604 Second Avenue, S.W., Rochester, MN 55902.

There are (as of March 1989) 114 ASDA-accredited Sleep Disorders Centers in the United States, and 27 accredited Laboratories for Sleep Related Breathing Disorders.

LABORATORY PROCEDURES

The laboratory procedures presently performed most often include polysomnography, the MSLT, and measurements of nocturnal penile tumescence for evaluation of erectile dysfunction.

POLYSOMNOGRAPHY

Polysomnography entails the recording of multiple physiological variables during sleep. A typical screening PSG might include the following variables:

- Horizontal and vertical eye movements
- Two electroencephalogram (EEG) channels for sleep staging (C3-A2 and C4-A1)
- Chin electromyogram (EMG)
- Left and right tibialis anterior EMG (separately if possible)
- EKG (for cardiac rate and rhythm)
- Intercostal EMG (helpful for ascertaining respiratory effort)
- Chest and abdominal strain gauges for measurement of respiratory excursion
- Nasal and oral thermistors for airflow
- Ear oximeter for oxygen saturation

This set of physiological variables would permit assessment of sleep stage, sleep respiration, cardiac rate and rhythm, and presence of periodic limb movements of sleep (nocturnal myoclonus). Patients with possible nocturnal seizures may require an additional 8–12 or more EEG channels, perhaps with video monitoring. Patients with sleep-related breathing disorders may be studied using additional measurements to provide a greater clarification of respiratory status, including precise measurements of quantified air exchange, esophageal pressure, and expired air CO_2. Patients who are suspected of gastroesophageal reflux may be studied using esophageal pH sensors.

Most PSG recordings are obtained on multichannel polygraphs with hand scoring of the paper records. Improvements in computerized data recording and analysis systems promise automation of these labor-intensive tasks in the future.

Polysomnographic examinations are normally conducted at night, but recordings may be obtained during the day in shiftworkers. The patient is instructed to report to the laboratory about 1½ hours before his or her normal bedtime to give the technician time to apply the necessary electrodes and transducers. The patient then retires, and, following necessary calibrations, the lights are turned out and the patient is allowed to sleep. Recording times may vary, but they typically last about 7½ to 8 hours.

MULTIPLE SLEEP LATENCY TEST

A MSLT is a test performed in the sleep laboratory that is designed to quantify the nature and degree of daytime sleepiness in patients complaining of EDS (6). The patient is given five opportunities to sleep. These five naps are spaced across the day at 2-hour intervals beginning at 10:00 A.M. The patients are polysomnographically monitored with at least an EEG, an electro-oculogram (EOG), and an EMG, so that wakefulness and the various stages of sleep may be defined. The mean sleep latency (MSL) (i.e., the average for all five tests of the time from the beginning of the test to sleep onset) and the presence of Stage REM sleep are noted. Because sleep deprivation can directly lead to EDS and an abnormally short mean sleep latency on the MSLT, this test should be performed the day following a nocturnal PSG. This will ensure that the patient had adequate sleep the preceding night. In addition, because this test should be done in a drug-free state, a drug screen is often necessary to rule out drug use.

Studies have defined normative data for the MSLT in various age groups. Pathological sleepiness is indicated by an MSL of 5 minutes or less. Normal alertness is confirmed by an MSL of greater than 12 to 13 minutes. The range between 5 and 12 minutes is a "gray zone" that can represent EDS from a variety of causes. The presence of Stage REM sleep within 10 minutes of sleep onset in two or more naps can help differentiate narcolepsy from other causes of pathological sleepiness.

NOCTURNAL PENILE TUMESCENCE

Nocturnal penile tumescence measures penile erections during sleep to help in the differential diagnosis of organic versus psychogenic impotence. This is primarily a urological or psychiatric diagnostic procedure and is not covered further in this volume.

HOW TO USE A SLEEP DISORDERS CENTER

As a rule of thumb, we believe *all patients complaining of EDS should be studied polysomnographically*. The exceptions would be those cases in which a simple and clearcut cause is apparent upon clinical evaluation (e.g., drug or sedative use and/or abuse, depression in adolescents), *and* the EDS resolves upon treatment of the underlying cause.

In the sleep-related breathing disorders, a nocturnal PSG is essential for determining the type and severity of the disorder, and followup recordings may be required in some cases to assess adequacy of treatment. It is often advisable to consider an MSLT along with a PSG on the initial recording. Some patients with EDS and symptoms strongly suggestive of a sleep-related breathing disorder may have the breathing disorder confirmed by a PSG, but their failure to respond appropriately to treatment ultimately leads to the additional diagnosis of narcolepsy, a diagnosis which was missed by failing to do an MSLT during the initial evaluation.

Even though narcolepsy can be diagnosed in the office based upon clinical symptoms (EDS with cataplexy is pathognomonic of narcolepsy), a PSG can identify other sleep-related problems, such as breathing disorders or myoclonus, that can influence treatment response. An MSLT can give some indication of REM pressure by the number of sleep-onset REM periods, their duration, and their degree of phasic activity. Equally important, stimulant abusers can become quite proficient in mimicking the symptoms of narcolepsy in order to obtain medications; they cannot, however, easily go undetected with an MSLT.

The parasomnias rarely require a PSG for their diagnosis, which is usually made on the basis of clinical history. It is hard to be certain that a parasomnia event will occur during the PSG; thus this procedure is usually not cost-effective in this case.

With the insomnias the situation is not quite as clear. In those cases where periodic leg movements (nocturnal myoclonus) or apnea is suspected on clinical grounds, a PSG is required for proper diagnosis. This procedure can be helpful in other cases as well. In a study of 128 patients with chronic insomnia, Jacobs et al. (7) found that in 49% of the patients a PSG added to, refuted, or failed to support an initial clinical impression. A recent study in our laboratory found the PSG to be useful in demonstrating unsuspected nocturnal myoclonus and apnea in patients thought to have chronic psychophysiological insomnia (8).

An important question is whether a single night's recording in the Sleep Disorders Center is sufficiently representative of the patient's disorder to result in an accurate diagnosis. That is, how much does sleep pathology vary night to night? It has long been noted that there is a "first-night effect" in sleep laboratory recordings. Subjects generally sleep better the second night, with less time awake, more restful sleep, more REM and Stage 3–Stage 4 sleep, and possibly shorter REM latencies. Similarly, sleep pathology may demonstrate night-to-night variability (9). Recordings of two or three nights, while perhaps ideal, are generally impractical because of both costs and patient compliance. Recordings are both expensive and tedious from the patient's standpoint. It is probably impractical, with today's technology, to routinely obtain a multiple-night diagnostic recording.

A single night's recording, to the extent it errs, will likely err in a conservative direction—it may miss diagnosing some (usually borderline) conditions, but it will likely not overdiagnose. Both apneas and periodic leg movements in the elderly have been shown to vary night by night, but this occurs predominantly in those cases that were marginal in severity. Severe cases are less likely to be missed on a single night's recording. A long REM latency the first night (not suggestive of a major affective disorder) is unlikely to be followed by a very short REM latency the second night (suggestive of a major affective disorder). On the other hand, a very short REM latency the first night is suggestive of a major affective disorder, irrespective of the second night's REM latency.

As with all laboratory tests the findings must be interpreted in the context of the entire clinical presentation. Stringent criteria (e.g., believing that a myoclonic index of <5 per hour assures no periodic leg movement problem) should not be applied automatically. Borderline laboratory values must be interpreted with caution, not by hard and fast rules. Similarly, it is important not to routinely refer all patients with sleep complaints to the Sleep Disorders Center for an all-night recording, and then use the findings from that study as a hard and fast diagnosis in the absence of a comprehensive evaluation. Patients with significant depression may also have marginal myoclonus and normal REM latencies. A polysomnographic report of a myoclonic index of 7 per hour, with a normal REM latency, in an insomniac but clinically depressed patient should not lead to an exclusive diagnosis of periodic leg movements, missing the depression.

■ REFERENCES

1. Bixler EO, Kales A, Soldatos CR, et al: Prevalence of sleep disorders in the Los Angeles metropolitan area. Am J Psychiatry 136:1257–1262, 1979
2. Association of Sleep Disorders Centers: Diagnostic classification of sleep and arousal disorders. Sleep 2:1–137, 1979 (reproduction with permission of Raven Press, New York)
3. Soldatos CR, Kales JD, Tan T, et al: Classification of sleep disorders. Psychiatr Annals 17:454–458, 1987
4. American Sleep Disorders Association, Diagnostic Classification Steering Committee (Thorpy MJ, Chair): International Classification of Sleep Disorders, Diagnostic and Coding Manual, draft outline, 1989
5. American Psychiatric Association: Diagnostic and Statistical Manual of Mental Disorders, Third Edition–Revised. Washington, DC, American Psychiatric Association, 1987
6. Richardson G, Carskadon M, Flagg W, et al: Excessive daytime sleepiness in man: multiple sleep latency measurements in narcoleptics vs. control subjects. Electroencephalogr Clin Neurophysiol 34:621–627, 1987
7. Jacobs EA, Reynolds CF, Kupfer DJ, et al: The role of polysomnography in the differential diagnosis of chronic insomnia. Am J Psychiatry 145:346–349, 1988
8. Reite M, Higgs L, Reed N: Polysomnographic findings in chronic psychophysiological insomnia. Sleep Research 18:293, 1989
9. Mosko SS, Dickel MJ, Ashorst J: Night to night variability in sleep apnea and sleep-related periodic leg movements in the elderly. Sleep 11:340–348, 1988

■ ADDITIONAL READING

Guilleminault C (ed): Sleeping and Waking Disorders: Indications and Techniques. Menlo Park, CA, Addison-Wesley, 1982

2 SLEEP PHYSIOLOGY AND PATHOLOGY

■ SLEEP ARCHITECTURE

Wakefulness in the typical adult is accompanied by a low-voltage fast scalp-recorded EEG, with frequencies usually above 8 Hz and amplitudes in the vicinity of 50 μV or less. The most prominent EEG rhythm of quiet relaxed wakefulness is the alpha rhythm, seen over the back of the head when the eyes are closed. Alpha rhythm consists of rhythmical 8- to 12-Hz activity, usually about 50 μV in amplitude. This rhythm disappears when the eyes are opened (called alpha blocking) or during times of visual imagery. In this section, illustrations of polygraph recordings during wakefulness, including an EEG, an EOG (eye movement), and an EMG (chin muscle activity), are compared to those of several sleep stages.

Figure 2-1 illustrates an awake record, with prominent alpha activity. The transition from wakefulness to sleep—normally Stage 1 non-REM sleep—is indicated by the appearance in the EEG of slower 5- to 7-Hz theta activity of generally low voltage (Figure 2-2). The subject is not responsive at this point, but can be easily aroused. After a few minutes the typical subject transitions into Stage 2 sleep (Figure 2-3), characterized by additional EEG slowing and the appearance of sleep spindles and K complexes. Spindles are short (usually <1 second) bursts of 12- to 14-Hz activity recorded over high central regions that wax and wane in amplitude—thus the term "spindle." They may be generated in or controlled by activity in midline thalamic nuclei, such as the centrum medianum. K complexes are large (high voltage), sharp wave complexes, often followed by spindle bursts, that are maximally seen over high central and central-parietal regions. They are thought to represent a type of EEG "evoked response" triggered by external or internal stimuli, and may also have as their source deeper brain structures.

Stage 3 and Stage 4 sleep usually follow Stage 2 and are characterized by increased slowing and increased amplitude of

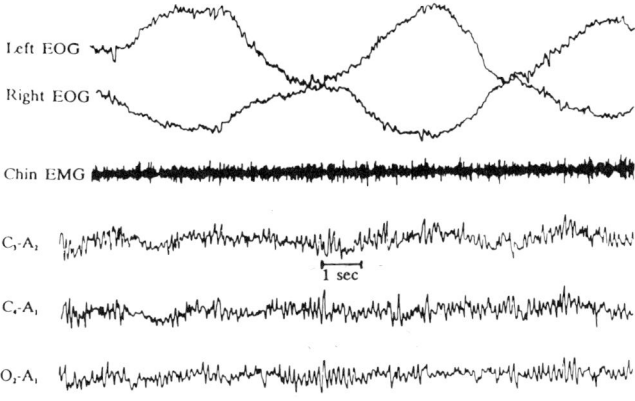

FIGURE 2-1. **Wakefulness.**

This state characterized by prominent alpha activity in the EEG, relatively high chin muscle activity in the EMG, and slow rolling eye movements in the EOG. C_3 = left high central EEG; C_4 = right high central EEG; A_2 = right ear; A_1 = left ear; O_2 = right occipital EEG.

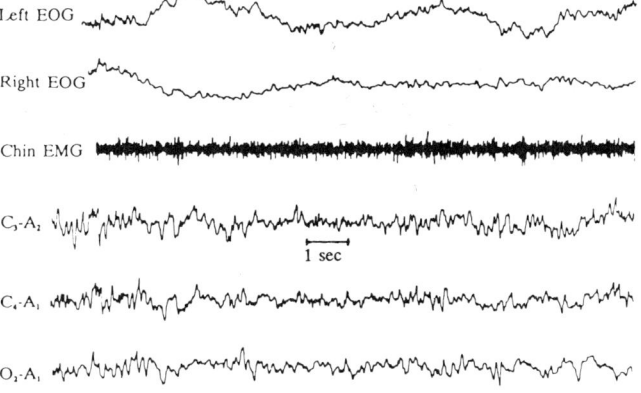

FIGURE 2-2. **Stage 1 sleep.**

Theta activity predominates in the EEG, and there is relatively high chin muscle activity in the EMG, and occasionally slow eye movements in the EOG.

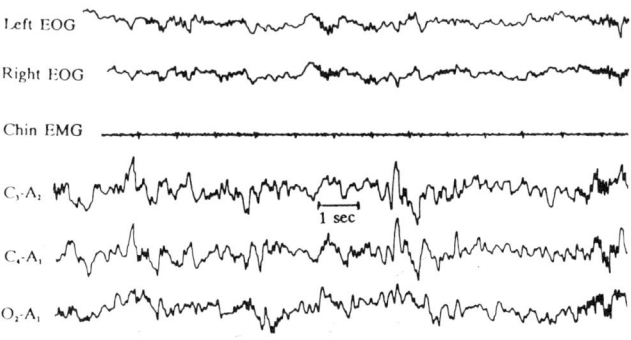

FIGURE 2-3. **Stage 2 sleep.**
K complexes and sleep spindles appear in the EEG. The EMG is low voltage, and there is EEG activity in the EOG leads.

the EEG. Stage 3 sleep contains between 20% and 50% of high-voltage (>75 μV), slow (<2 Hz) delta activity (Figure 2-4), and Stage 4 sleep contains >50% slow delta activity (Figure 2-5). Sleep spindles are more difficult to see in Stage 3 and Stage 4 sleep, but may still be present. Stage 3 and Stage 4 sleep are often grouped together as "delta sleep."

After the typical young adult has been asleep (in non-REM or "slow wave sleep") for about 90 minutes, the EEG again has lower voltage and becomes relatively fast. The subject remains asleep, but the eyes can be seen moving beneath the closed lids. Consequently, this stage of sleep is called "rapid eye movement," or "REM" sleep (Figure 2-6). If awakened during this stage the subject will most often report a dream. The time period from sleep onset (i.e., Stage 1) to the onset of the first REM period is called the "REM latency," which has important differential diagnostic implications, being shorter than normal in many adult depressed patients, and occasionally in narcoleptic patients. REM latency tends to decrease with advancing age, but as a rule of thumb, nocturnal REM latency of less than 60 minutes in an adult should be considered abnormally short and suggestive of possible narcolepsy, a major affective disorder, or another sleep abnormality.

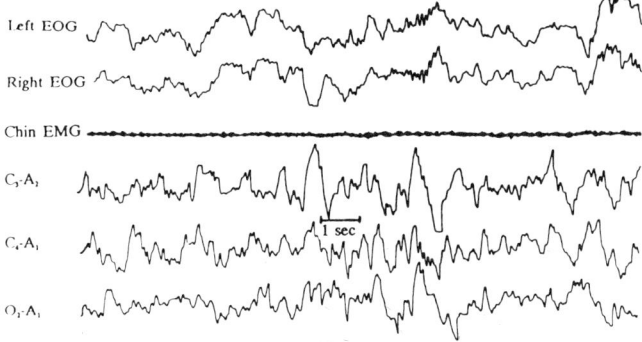

FIGURE 2-4. **Stage 3 sleep.**
Slow, high-voltage delta activity comprises 20–50% of the EEG activity. Chin muscle activity (EMG) is low, and EEG activity is seen in the EOG leads.

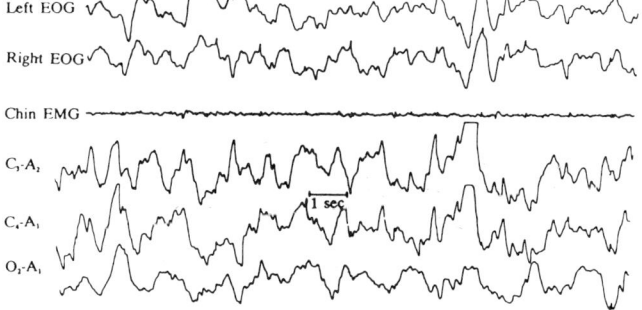

FIGURE 2-5. **Stage 4 sleep.**
Slow, high-voltage delta activity comprises greater than 50% of the EEG activity. The chin muscle activity (EMG) is low voltage, and EEG activity is seen in the EOG leads.

REM sleep is often described as having "tonic" and "phasic" components. Tonic REM activity consists of the generally low-voltage activated EEG, with a general decrease in skeletal muscle tone. Phasic activity includes eye movement bursts, episodic increases in middle ear muscle activity, and episodic EMG

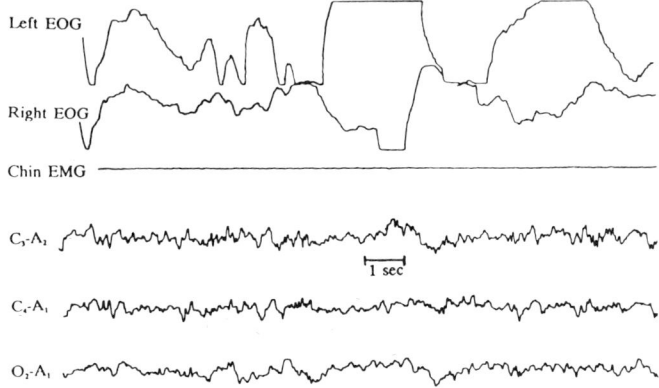

FIGURE 2-6. **REM sleep.**
This sleep stage is characterized by fast, low-voltage activity in the EEG. Chin muscle activity (EMG) is virtually absent, and rapid eye movement is seen in the EOG leads.

bursts (on the suppressed background). The latter have been suggestively correlated with dream content.

REM periods typically end with brief arousals and/or transitions into Stage 2 sleep once again. The completion of the period from Stage 1 through Stage 4 to REM sleep is considered to represent a "sleep cycle," and a night's sleep is usually made up of several (usually about three to five) such consecutive cycles. (A detailed presentation of the scoring of sleep stages can be found in the manual prepared by Rechtschaffen and Kales (1).

During the time course of a normal night the nature of the sleep cycles changes considerably. Stage 3 and Stage 4 sleep are usually only seen during the first part of the night, and are usually not found in the sleep cycles occurring, for example, in the early morning hours. Sleep disorders associated with Stage 3 and Stage 4 sleep (the parasomnias such as sleepwalking and night terrors) tend to occur preferentially early in the sleep period when most Stage 3 and Stage 4 sleep occurs. REM sleep periods (except in patients with depression or a major affective disorder) usually are shorter and have fewer eye movements (phasic activity) early in the night, becoming longer, with more phasic activity, as the night progresses. And accordingly, sleep disorders associated with REM sleep (nightmares and certain sleep-related breathing disorders) may be more pronounced later in the sleep period when most REM sleep occurs. After a long night's sleep, especially, for example, on a weekend morning when we might tend to "sleep in," the sleep cycles just before awakening might include only Stage 2 sleep and REM sleep in equal proportions, and therefore we are more likely to awaken from a dream.

The cyclic nature of normal sleep in a typical adult, as well as the tendency for different stages to predominate at different times, is illustrated in Figure 2-7.

■ ONTOGENY OF SLEEP ARCHITECTURE AND SLEEP PATTERNS

EEG patterns and sleep pattern distribution change dramatically from birth to adulthood. The newborn infant, who exhibits a less well-organized EEG, spends approximately 50% of sleep time in REM sleep (premature infants spend even more—up to 80% at 30 weeks gestational age), with REM percent approaching adult levels during early childhood. Newborns typically have REM

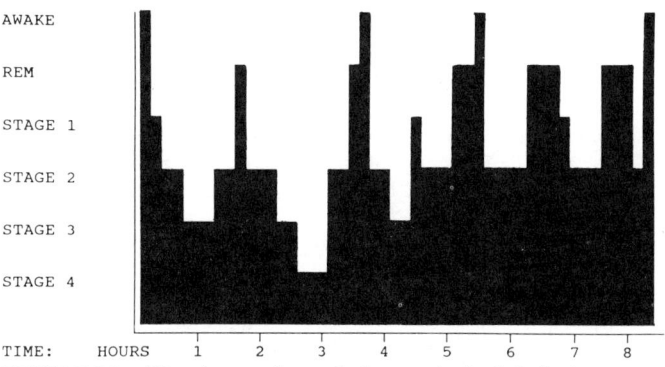

FIGURE 2-7. **The sleep-wake cycle in a typical adult during one night.**

Most Stage 3 and Stage 4 sleep is seen during the first half of the night. REM periods become longer as the night progresses.

onset sleep periods, shifting to adult non-REM onset sleep periods by about 4 months of age. Newborn sleep is generally about equally divided into "active" (REM) sleep and "quiet" sleep—the forerunner of later-developing Stage 2, Stage 3, and Stage 4 sleep. At birth, and in premature infants, the EEG of quiet sleep is characterized by a burst-suppression-type or a "trace-alternant"-type pattern. Stage 2 and delta (Stage 3 and Stage 4) sleep can usually be identified by about 3 months of age.

At birth, as every parent knows, a 24-hour sleep-wake pattern is not present—sleep tends to be randomly interspersed throughout the 24-hour period. In most infants consolidation of sleep during the night and wakefulness during the day begin to be seen at about 16 weeks of age, although there is considerable individual variability.

Total sleep time diminishes with age, ranging from 16 hours per 24 hours at birth, to about 9 hours at age 6, about 8 hours at age 12, and typically about 7½ hours in adulthood. REM latency in latency-age children is about 2 hours. The first sleep period in late latency and in the early teens usually contains a sustained period of deep Stage 3–Stage 4 sleep from which it may be quite difficult to awaken the child, and during which parasomnias may occur.

During adult life a decrease in Stage 3 and Stage 4 sleep is usually noted, but this may primarily be because of a decrease in amplitude of EEG slow waves so that they are no longer formally scorable as Stage 3 or Stage 4 sleep, rather than because of a diminution in the presence of slow activity per se. Young adults may have 25% of sleep time in Stage 3 and Stage 4 sleep; adults at age 50–60 may have 10% or less of sleep in these stages.

■ PHYSIOLOGY AND NEUROPHYSIOLOGY OF SLEEP

Sleep—both REM and non-REM—is an active process. We do not go to sleep only because of a decrease in sensory input, but rather because there is both a decrease in sensory stimulation and an increase in activity in those brain systems whose activity promotes the sleep state. Arousal is maintained by the activity of the brain system known as the ascending reticular activating system, or ARAS. This system, identified initially by neurophysiological studies in animals, is composed predominantly of small neurons with many interconnecting fibers (therefore "reticular") that surround the center of the neuraxis beginning in the spinal cord and ascending into the diencephalon (therefore "ascending"). When the ARAS is electrically stimulated, it arouses or alerts (therefore "activating") the animal. If the ARAS is lesioned, either experimentally or accidentally, the subject (animal or human) may become somnolent and difficult to arouse. Activity in the ARAS must diminish for sleep to occur. But in addition, activity in the midbrain raphe and basal forebrain sleep-inducing systems must increase at the same time if sleep (non-REM or slow wave) is to ensue and be maintained.

REM sleep is also actively triggered, but by neuronal systems deep in the brain, in the region of the pontine tegmentum. Hobson and McCarley (2) have suggested that so-called giant FTG (large cells found in the field tegmentum gigantocellularis) are important in this triggering action. Cholinergic mechanisms seem to be important in turning REM sleep systems on, and monoaminergic mechanisms in turning it off. These systems may also control the various other manifestations of REM sleep, including eye movements, postural atonia, the general EEG arousal (low voltage, fast activity), and the unique EEG waves such as "PGO spikes" or "sawtooth waves" that accompany REM sleep. Probably the most important issue here is that REM sleep is triggered by systems deep in the brain stem area that can project both up and down, and so control the multiple physiological accompaniments of the REM state.

SLEEP PHYSIOLOGY

Autonomic activity, such as cardiac and respiratory rate, is usually somewhat slower and more regular during non-REM sleep than during wakefulness. Skeletal muscle EMG similarly diminishes slightly as the sleeping subject relaxes. During REM sleep, however, autonomic activity can become quite variable and highly irregular, with large and rapid changes in cardiac and respiratory rate and blood pressure accompanying REM sleep. Most deaths occur in the early morning hours when the propensity for REM sleep is highest; some have suggested there may be a relationship between the variable physiology accompanying REM and the increased incidence of death in vulnerable individuals.

Body temperature regulation temporarily ceases during REM sleep, and we become for a short time essentially poikilothermic animals. Body temperature also, of course, has a prominent 24-hour "circadian" rhythm, tending to be lowest in the early morning hours and highest in the midday. The probability of REM sleep occurring is highest when body temperature is lowest, and the peak of REM sleep propensity is coincidental with the rising slope of body temperature, just after it reaches its lowest point (3).

REM sleep is also frequently accompanied by penile erections in males (and clitoral erections in females). This normal component of REM state physiology provides a valuable tool in the differential diagnosis of psychogenic and organic impotence. A nocturnal polysomnogram accompanied by monitoring of nocturnal penile tumescence is highly recommended in the evaluation of erectile dysfunction, and certainly before the consideration of penile reconstructive procedures. Lack of erection during REM sleep is probably not conclusive evidence of an organic disorder, however, because there is evidence that psychological status may influence REM erections.

CIRCADIAN PHYSIOLOGY AND SLEEP

Like most living organisms, humans exhibit prominent daily, or circadian ("about a day"), biological rhythms, which have important implications for sleep disorders. The body's major internal circadian oscillator is manifest in the rhythm of body temperature and serum cortisol. Body temperature is lowest in the early morning hours prior to awakening, and serum cortisol reaches its lowest point around the time of sleep onset, increasing before awakening in the morning. Body temperature and serum cortisol rhythms reflect the activity of a master oscillator, probably located in the suprachiasmatic nucleus of the hypothalamus.

The normal sleep-wake rhythm is also a 24-hour rhythm that is normally synchronized to the circadian temperature and cortisol oscillator as outlined above, but that may become desynchronized, as for example during jet lag, when the sleep-wake rhythm is forced to a new time, with the circadian oscillator remaining on the original schedule until it has time to be reentrained to the new schedule.

Human subjects who live in caves or other environments without time cues will normally adopt a body temperature and sleep-wake rhythm of about 25 hours, not 24 hours. This suggests that the normal free-running circadian period of most body rhythms is closer to 25 hours than to 24, and that these rhythms must be "phase-advanced" about 1 hour each day to stay in synchronization with the 24-hour rhythm of the sun. It is physiologically difficult, however, to phase-advance rhythms much more than an extra hour each day (2 hours total), and west-to-east travel requires phase advancement (e.g., sleep onset time becomes earlier). Phase delay, however, as in east-to-west travel, takes advantage of the body's free-running 25-hour period, which means adaptation is more rapid; in addition, it appears somewhat easier for the body's rhythms to phase-delay than to phase-advance. Some individuals seem unable to phase-advance sleep rhythms and may develop circadian rhythm-based sleep disorders (see Chapter 3).

Light is a major synchronizer of circadian rhythms, and recently it has become apparent that, as in most other organisms, circadian rhythms in humans can be reset by appropriately timed exposure to bright light (4). The phase response curve (PRC) is an experimentally generated curve that plots how the timing of light exposure affects circadian rhythm timing. PRCs have been developed for many organisms, but only recently has a suggestive PRC been outlined for humans. This PRC suggests that exposure to bright light immediately before or shortly after onset of the sleep period (i.e., typically in the late evening) will tend to delay the circadian system, whereas exposure late in the sleep period or immediately after awakening (i.e., early morning) will tend to advance the circadian system. The human PRC may provide useful information for timing the use of bright-light exposure as a therapeutic modality for treatment of circadian rhythm disorders (see Chapter 3). It is not yet clear how intense the light must be to serve as a synchronizer of the circadian system. However, studies using intensities of 2,500 lux or greater have been successful.

Growth hormone release is generally associated with the onset of Stage 3 and Stage 4 slow wave sleep in adults. Unlike cortisol, however, growth hormone is locked to the sleep-wake rhythm, and if sleep does not occur, growth hormone is not released. Similarly, if sleep is suddenly changed to a new time period, growth hormone release will remain locked to Stage 3 and Stage 4 sleep at the new time. The growth hormone–sleep relationship is not seen in early infancy (under 3 months) and tends to diminish or disappear in the elderly.

Several other hormones exhibit circadian rhythms. Prolactin secretion, like growth hormone secretion, is also linked to sleep, increasing about 60–90 minutes after sleep onset, and peaking shortly before awakening. Luteinizing hormone levels rise during sleep in early pubescent subjects but not in adults. This relationship has been used to identify the onset of puberty before secondary sexual characteristics appear.

Melatonin secretion is also increased during sleep, but can be suppressed by exposure to bright light, and appears to be related more to the light-dark cycle than to the sleep-wake cycle.

DREAMING

The dream is that mental content that accompanies the REM state. While dreams may indeed be "the royal road to the unconscious" in the hands of a psychotherapist, there is no good evidence for any general form of dream symbolism (such as the snake being a symbol for the penis), nor can dreams predict the future. Rather, the vivid hallucinatory imagery seems to be a by-product—almost an epiphenomenon—of the heightened state of CNS arousal accompanying the REM state, with the dream perhaps representing the effort of the neocortex to make sense out of the essentially random and chaotic input being received from highly activated lower brain centers. It remains to be seen if the specifics of the way in which the neocortex tries to "make sense" in the form of the dream have a predictable and perhaps psychodynamically generalizable form.

Lucid dreams are dreams in which the dreamer is in the REM state but knows the dream to be a dream—and may even to some extent be able to control the dream experience. Lucid dreams may occur predominantly during REM sleep with greater-than-normal alpha EEG content (5).

Nightmares are particularly vivid and often frightening dreams that arise during the normal course of REM sleep. Nightmares must be differentiated from *night terrors*, which are disorders of arousal from non-REM sleep (see Chapter 5).

HUMORAL CONTROL OF SLEEP

There has long been interest in whether some specific factor or substance that triggers or influences sleep might be produced in the brain. A peptide termed delta sleep-inducing peptide, or Factor S, may represent several naturally occurring peptide substances, including several muramyl peptides, and appears to increase slow wave sleep in animals (6, 7).

SLEEP AND IMMUNE FUNCTION

Sleep appears closely related to immunological function. The onset of slow wave sleep especially has been found to be associated with increases in plasma interleukin-1 activity, and with increases in lymphocyte response to mitogen stimulation (8). It is possible that sleep deprivation may be accordingly associated with impairment in immune function. Another peptide, interferon alpha-A, also involved in immune function, whose level is increased during certain viral infections that are accompanied by feelings of depression and malaise, has been shown to shorten REM latency (9), a phenomenon also associated with major depression in humans.

FUNCTIONS OF SLEEP

Sleep appears to serve a restorative function for the organism. In fact, some have suggested that non-REM sleep serves a restorative function for the body, and REM sleep, for the brain. Limited evidence directly supports such theories, with perhaps the best evidence yet available being that experienced by each person each morning after a good night of sleep. Growth hormone and other anabolic hormones such as prolactin, testosterone, and luteinizing hormone have sleep-dependent secretion rhythms, tending to support the restorative function theory. Other theories consider sleep as a time of energy conservation, or postulate that sleep serves an adaptive function in promoting survival. It remains for future research to determine which of these theories can best be empirically supported.

SLEEP DEPRIVATION

Animals that are totally deprived of sleep for prolonged periods (up to 30 days) will eventually die with general debilitation and multiple organ failure (10). Humans have experimentally tolerated up to about 10 days of acute total sleep deprivation without evidence of serious prolonged consequences. Individuals undergoing total sleep deprivation have much greater difficulty maintaining wakefulness during their normal sleep periods than during their normal wake periods. These individuals often develop "microsleeps," consisting of brief (a few seconds) epochs of slow wave activity in the EEG. They can usually arouse themselves, with effort (and perhaps help), to perform well on psychomotor performance tasks for short periods.

The deleterious effects, if any, of chronic partial sleep deprivation remain to be elucidated.

■ REFERENCES

1. Rechtschaffen A, Kales A: A Manual of Standardized Terminology. Techniques and Scoring System for Sleep Stages of Human Sleep Subjects. Washington, DC, U.S. Government Printing Office, 1968
2. Hobson JA, McCarley RW: The brain as a dream state generator: an activation-synthesis hypothesis of the dream process. Am J Psychiatry 134:1335–1368, 1977
3. Czeisler CA, Zimmerman JC, Ronda JM, et al: Timing of REM sleep is coupled to the circadian rhythm of body temperature in man. Sleep 2:329–346, 1980
4. Czeisler CA, Allan JA, Strogatz SH, et al: Bright light resets the human circadian pacemaker independent of the timing of the sleep-wake cycle. Science 233:667–671, 1986

5. Ogilvie RD, Hunt HT, Tyson PD, et al: Lucid dreaming and alpha activity: a preliminary report. Percept Mot Skills 55:795–808, 1982
6. Krueger JM: Muramy: peptide enhancement of slow wave sleep. Methods Find Exp Clin Pharmacol 8:105–110, 1986
7. Susic V, Masirevic G, Totic S: The effects of delta-sleep-inducing peptide (DSIP) on wakefulness and sleep patterns in the cat. Brain Res 414:262–270, 1987
8. Moldofsky H, Lue FA, Eisen J, et al: The relationship of interleukin-1 and immune functions to sleep in humans. Psychosom Med 48:309–318, 1986
9. Reite M, Laudenslager M, Jones J, et al: Interferon decreases REM latency. Biol Psychiatry 22:104–107, 1987
10. Rechtschaffen A, Bergmann BM, Everson CA, et al: Sleep deprivation in the rat: X. Integration and discussion of the findings. Sleep 12:68–87, 1989

■ ADDITIONAL READINGS

Anch AM, Browman CP, Mitler MM, et al (eds): Sleep: A Scientific Perspective. Englewood Cliffs, NJ, Prentice-Hall, 1988
Hobson JA: The Dreaming Brain. New York, Basic Books, 1988
Kleitman N: Sleep and Wakefulness. Chicago, IL, University of Chicago Press, 1963
Parkes JD: Sleep and Its Disorders. London, WB Saunders, 1985

TRANSIENT AND CHRONIC INSOMNIAS

The Disorders of Initiating or Maintaining Sleep (DIMS) are usually grouped as either transient or chronic.

■ TRANSIENT INSOMNIAS

Transient insomnias (e.g., 3 weeks or less) are ubiquitous. Most individuals experience short-term trouble with sleep latency or sleep maintenance at times of stress, excitement, or anticipation, during an illness, or at high altitudes. Such problems rarely come to the attention of the clinician in the early stages. These symptoms can nonetheless be decreased, and daytime functioning improved, if certain guidelines are followed. Stress-related insomnia, or temporary trouble sleeping in response to excitement or worry (e.g., anticipating a trip or a forthcoming examination), may appropriately be treated with a night or two of a short-half-life benzodiazepine (e.g., triazolam [Halcion] 0.125 to 0.25 mg hs). This need not be taken in anticipation of trouble sleeping but can be deferred until the patient has been unable to get to sleep for 30–60 minutes. The principles of good sleep hygiene (described later in this chapter) are important as well. It is important that pharmacological intervention be seen as short-term and symptomatic. The appropriate treatment of a transient insomnia may prevent it from developing into a longer-term problem like chronic psychophysiological insomnia.

High-altitude insomnia is seen when most individuals suddenly go to higher altitudes. It frequently accompanies ski and mountain climbing trips. High-altitude insomnia results primarily from increases in sleep-related central apneas, and can be effectively diminished or prevented by several days of acetazolamide 250 mg bid or tid. A short-acting benzodiazepine such as triazolam 0.125–0.25 mg or temazepam 15 mg may also be useful for a night or two. This insomnia normally improves spontaneously after several days at the high altitude.

■ EVALUATION OF CHRONIC INSOMNIA

Insomnia is a complaint, DIMS a group of disorders. While the differential diagnosis and effective treatment of chronic insomnia can challenge the most skilled clinician, we have tried to outline a rational step-wise procedure to facilitate the efficient and accurate differential diagnosis of the majority of patients with complaints relating to insomnia. An accurate differential diagnosis is very important. A variety of different causes of insomnia can present in a very similar fashion, and the appropriate treatment for one may aggravate another. The clinician who does not systematically pursue a differential diagnosis will wind up with misdiagnoses, treatment failures, and dissatisfied patients.

While most DIMS patients have a presenting complaint of insomnia, it is important to realize that a substantial disturbance of nocturnal sleep can present as complaints of chronic fatigue, impaired daytime performance, and excessive daytime sleepiness (EDS), raising the question of a possible Disorders of Excessive Somnolence (DOES). A careful history should identify such patients, however, so that a more appropriate inquiry into nocturnal sleep habits and patterns can be undertaken. Similarly, a variety of medical disorders can result in insomnia complaints. These problem areas are dealt with separately in Chapter 6.

A detailed *sleep history* (see Chapter 1) is the first order of business with a chronic sleep complaint. Assuming the sleep history suggests a chronic DIMS, we then need to focus on the probable causes of the insomnia. The sleep history will include the type of insomnia problem (sleep onset, sleep maintenance, early awakening), when it began (childhood, recently, at time of major stress or life event), when it occurs (every night, weeknights only, at times of stress), what has been done when and by whom, previous response to treatment, and similar issues. Is there a family history? How does the insomnia impact daytime functioning? A sleep diary (see Chapter 1) kept for 1–2 weeks may be helpful in establishing the type, perceived severity, and periodicity of the insomnia.

At this point, the differential diagnosis is facilitated by a systematic approach such as outlined below, using the schematic decision tree illustrated in Figure 3-1.

Step 1. First one should inquire about and evaluate the presence of other medical conditions that may contribute to the insomnia. If appropriate, this inquiry may include a complete medical history and physical with appropriate laboratory tests. Special attention should be paid to evidence of endocrinopathies and to disorders associated with chronic pain. It should be remembered that the incidence of medical disorders accounting for sleep complaints increases with age. Also, a number of prescription drugs may result in insomnia complaints. (See Chapter 6 for a more detailed discussion of the relationship between medical disorders and sleep complaints.)

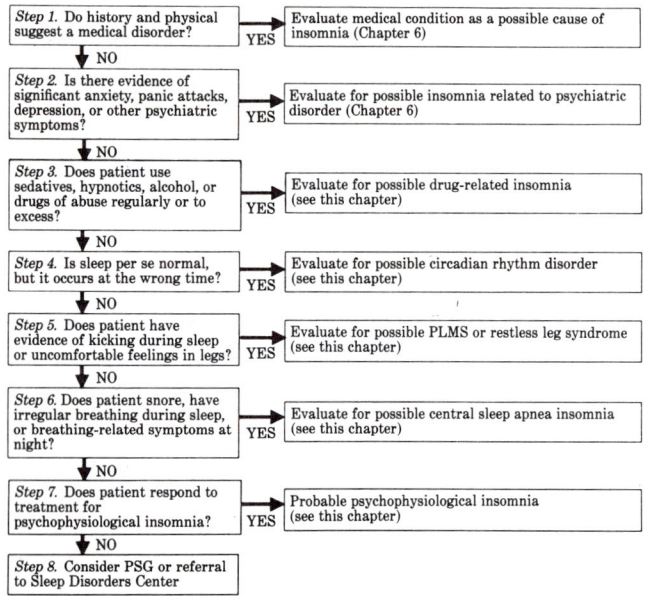

FIGURE 3-1. **Decision tree for differential diagnosis of chronic insomnia.**

Step 2. The presence of significant anxiety, dysphoric mood, or frank depression with sleep complaints should alert one to a possible psychiatric-related insomnia. Nocturnal panic attacks are a not infrequent cause of chronic insomnia, even in individuals who are not markedly anxious during the day or who do not experience typical panic episodes during the day. Accordingly, special attention should be paid to evidence of nocturnal arousals accompanied by autonomic symptoms such as tachycardia, rapid breathing, and the sense of anxiety or fearfulness. Insomnias related to psychiatric causes usually co-vary with the degree of psychiatric symptoms (see Chapter 6).

Step 3. A careful drug history will help identify patients who have used *sedatives or hypnotics*, including alcohol, nightly for many months to years in order to get to sleep. Similarly, a history of stimulant use or drug abuse may result in a sleep disorder. A history of chronic or excessive drug or alcohol use recounted by the patient, or, equally important, by the family member or friend, suggests that further workup in this area is required, as outlined below in the next section.

Step 4. Patients whose sleep is normal (i.e., they go to sleep easily at the right time for them and can sleep uninterrupted and feel rested if they get enough sleep) but whose sleep occurs at the wrong time, or at unusual hours (e.g., they cannot get to sleep until 4 A.M.), may be suffering from a *circadian rhythm disorder*, such as delayed sleep phase syndrome. These patients will usually present, however, with a chief complaint of insomnia (i.e., "I can't get to sleep until the night is almost over"). In these cases careful questioning is required to find out whether once asleep these patients do fine if allowed to sleep until they are ready to get up (e.g., noon), but they are chronically sleep-deprived if they must arise at 8 A.M. to get to work or school. (The circadian rhythm disorders are covered below in a later section of this chapter.)

Step 5. It is important to make careful inquiry into the possibility of restless leg syndrome or periodic limb movements of sleep (PLMS) (also called nocturnal myoclonus). Restless legs, characterized by uncomfortable sensations in the calves at sleep onset, requiring the patient to get up and walk them out, is not a sleep disorder per se but can significantly interfere with the patient's getting to sleep. PLMS are usually not perceived by the patient but may be perceived by the bed partner as kicking movements during the night. Sometimes patients will say their bedclothes are in disarray or kicked onto the floor in the morning. Rarely, leg jerks may be noted while resting in the waking state or while napping in a chair. Restless leg syndrome or suspicion of a PLMS disorder requires a more comprehensive sleep workup, including possibly a polysomnogram (PSG), as detailed later in this chapter. The initial history and evaluation may fail to suggest evidence of a PLMS disorder. Not infrequently, such problems are found only on a PSG, after the patient has failed to respond to treatment for a presumed diagnosis of psychophysiological insomnia.

Step 6. Central apnea is an occasional cause of chronic insomnia, especially in the older patient. (Insomnia secondary to sleep apnea is discussed in detail later in this chapter.) Inquiry should be made as to whether the patient has had any subjective sense of trouble getting his or her breath or feeling like his or her breathing is interfered with, especially in the transition from wakefulness to sleep. The bed partner should be asked if the patient has irregular breathing or pauses in his or her breathing during sleep. Snoring is another clue. As with PLMS, central apnea-related insomnia may be missed on the initial workup and may only become apparent on a PSG after failure to respond to other treatment. Fortunately, this insomnia is uncommon. The more common obstructive apneas typically present as EDS, not insomnia (see Chapter 4 for discussion of these sleep-related breathing disorders).

Step 7. Finally, having ruled out the foregoing causes, one is left with the possibility of chronic psychophysiological insomnia. This is not only a diagnosis of exclusion, however, for there are a number of characteristic symptoms and complaints that raise the index of suspicion for this diagnosis, such as a history of insomnia, usually at sleep onset, beginning during a time of stress and then being aggravated by a fear of not being able to sleep, even after the initial stress is resolved. Patients with this syndrome often sleep better when not in their own bed (e.g., while on vacation). Statistically, psychophysiological insomnia (discussed in detail later in this chapter) and psychiatric-related insomnia are the categories that account for the majority of chronic insomnia complaints.

Several other less common types of chronic insomnia, including childhood onset insomnia and REM interruption insomnia, may also fall into this last group by the process of exclusion. These less common disorders are part of the differential diagnosis of psychophysiological insomnia and are discussed in more detail later in this chapter.

It is important to remember that more than one cause of chronic insomnia may be present. A patient may, for example, have both a chronic psychophysiological insomnia and a PLMS-related disorder, or anxiety, depression, etc. Thus a complete differential diagnosis should be gone through for each patient; we should not stop when a first probable cause is encountered.

Step 8. If the patient fails to respond to treatment for psychophysiological insomnia, a more comprehensive evaluation is likely indicated, which might include a referral to a Sleep Disorders Center.

■ INSOMNIA SECONDARY TO SUBSTANCE ABUSE AND DRUG DEPENDENCY

PRESENTING COMPLAINTS

- Chronic insomnia in a substance abuse patient
- Chronic insomnia in a patient who has been using a sedative-hypnotic agent on a regular basis for many months to several years
- Insomnia associated with sudden withdrawal of a benzodiazepine or other sedative-hypnotic agent

CLINICAL PRESENTATION

Sleep-related concerns about substance abuse can be divided into three basic phases: *active abuse*, *initial withdrawal*, and *protracted withdrawal* (greater than 2 weeks after use).

Active alcohol users will frequently complain of many awakenings during the night. The alcohol abuser may even "treat" these awakenings with repeated alcohol administration. After the initial sedation, sleep will tend to be unrefreshing because of the fragmentation and numerous arousals caused by the alcohol. These characteristics are similar to those for abuse of other sedative agents. Active *cocaine* abusers will frequently report that they do not sleep at all throughout much of the week and then may have a day or two when they "crash" to get a few hours of sleep. This may be followed by a return to the stimulant use until the user needs to "crash" again. It is not uncommon for the chronic cocaine or amphetamine user to report many years of sleeping only on weekends or Sundays.

The withdrawal phase in most substance abuse patients is a period of serious insomnia, with the patient sleeping 1–4 hours per night for a number of days. REM rebound (an increase in REM sleep following its long-term suppression by the use of the substance) is commonly present, possibly for up to 30 days. REM sleep during this period may be associated with anxiety dreams or nightmares, and frequent awakenings throughout the night. A high percentage of alcoholic patients will have severe depressive symptoms during the first 2 weeks after they have stopped using alcohol; about 75–80% of depressive symptoms will resolve with time. Stimulant users may go through an immediate period of hyperactivity; others will experience a hypersomnolent period with considerable lethargy. The withdrawal syndrome of hypersomnolence, fatigue, lethargy, and depression typically lasts for a period of about 1 week.

Most substance abuse patients will still be complaining of severe insomnia and secondary fatigue and irritability for many weeks after cessation of use. Alcoholic patients postwithdrawal may also exhibit a similar long-term insomnia or continued sleep fragmentation, and also can exhibit symptoms of postwithdrawal hypomanic behavior, in which case moderate insomnia may be accompanied by irritability, grandiosity, hyperactivity, and moderately elevated mood, which can often lead to poor planning for the future and high likelihood for relapse to alcoholism.

Chronic use of sedative-hypnotic agents, especially some of the older hypnotics, or alcohol, may induce a chronic sleep disturbance characterized as a *drug dependency insomnia*. Such patients often present when they are attempting to discontinue their medications. These patients may also be referred for treatment in the face of continuing escalation of the dose required to maintain hypnotic effectiveness. This condition should be suspected in any individual who gives a history of chronic, long-term sedative or alcohol consumption. Often history from a family member or friend is necessary to elicit this information. The insomnia is substantially aggravated by sudden decreases in drug dose. These types of sleep disturbances appear to be related to two perhaps different mechanisms: *drug dependency insomnia* and/or *drug withdrawal insomnia.*

Insomnia also frequently accompanies withdrawal from sedative agents, such as the benzodiazepines, that have been prescribed regularly in therapeutic doses for several weeks to months or longer. Insomnia complaints of this type are called "*rebound insomnia.*"

ETIOLOGY AND PATHOPHYSIOLOGY

Drug dependency insomnia appears in conjunction with chronic use of agents that have often been started either by a physician, in the case of most sedative-hypnotic agents, or by the patient, in the case of alcohol. Most (nonbenzodiazepine) sedative-hypnotic agents lose their effectiveness with time, often in 1–2 weeks, and continued use may lead to further sleep disruption of the type present initially that led to the drug being started in the first place. In addition, these agents (e.g., barbiturates, glutethimide) suppress REM sleep, which leads to a REM rebound following their withdrawal, with intense REM sleep frequently associated with frightening dreams or nightmares. Thus an insomnia condition initially treated with a hypnotic may return as the drug loses its effectiveness, with a tendency for the dose of the hypnotic to be further increased, only to be followed by persistent insomnia once again. Furthermore, attempts to terminate the drugs may lead to a marked aggravation of the insomnia; thus the insomnia becomes drug dependent.

There appears to be a degree of individual variability in vulnerability to the development of drug dependency insomnia. The pathophysiology is not clear, but in some cases it is thought that chronic administration of a sedative-hypnotic agent may result in a compensatory increase in activity of the reticular activating system, and possibly alterations in brain protein synthesis as well, leading to impaired sleep maintenance.

Withdrawal from benzodiazepine hypnotic agents, which may have been originally administered for other reasons such as anxiety, may be accompanied by a rebound insomnia, as well as a related condition, *rebound anxiety* (1). These conditions are sometimes difficult to separate from reemergence of the original symptoms of insomnia or anxiety for which the medication was originally prescribed. Symptoms appear soon (the next night) following the quick cessation of a regularly taken short-acting benzodiazepine compound such as triazolam, but may be delayed up to 2 weeks following the cessation of a long-acting compound such as diazepam or flurazepam (2). Drug withdrawal symptoms have been described after substituting a short-acting for a long-acting benzodiazepine (3). Rebound insomnia and anxiety are thought to result from supersensitivity of the benzodiazepine receptor, whose naturally occurring ligand has been replaced by the exogenously administered drug. Symptoms persist until the brain again produces the naturally occurring agents in sufficient amount or until receptors are sufficiently down-regulated. These conditions may represent a specific subset of the more general drug withdrawal syndrome.

LABORATORY STUDIES

In the case of drug dependency insomnia, polysomnography confirms disturbed sleep and often will demonstrate intrusion of fast activity into the slow or sleep background, resulting in a markedly abnormal sleep morphology. Sometimes this type of a pattern is called an alpha-delta sleep pattern, indicating an intrusion of faster alpha frequency activity (although not necessarily physiologically normal alpha activity) into the slow wave sleep background. (See Figure 6-1 for example of an alpha-delta sleep pattern.)

Polysomnographic abnormalities can persist from months to several years following cessation of the offending drug, during which time sleep complaints may also persist. The incidental findings of such a disturbed polysomnographic tracing in a patient complaining of chronic insomnia might lead to inquiries into whether the patient had in the past been utilizing sedative-hypnotic agents to excess, if this information had not already been elicited.

A PSG during withdrawal from REM-suppressant drugs will demonstrate REM rebound, with shorter REM latencies, increased REM time, and increased REM phasic activity.

DIFFERENTIAL DIAGNOSIS

Sleep disturbances following drug termination in substance abuse patients are to be expected, but consideration should be given to the presence of other possible coincidental causes of insomnia as well. Drug dependency insomnia and drug withdrawal insomnia are suspected on the basis of history of chronic use of sedative-hypnotic agents, perhaps initially started for insomnia, with persistent sleep complaints on high doses and marked worsening of sleep, including perhaps evidence of REM rebound with vivid or frightening dreams during periods of attempts to terminate or reduce the offending medications. Polysomnography is usually not required, but if performed it may demonstrate an alpha-delta-type slow wave sleep morphology (see Figure 6-1). Prominent EEG changes will alert the clinician to the possibility that withdrawal may be difficult, with persistent complaints of insomnia even after the offending medications have been terminated.

Differential diagnosis is complicated when multiple medications have been used together, often for long periods of time. The best approach is usually to slowly eliminate as many of these medications as possible so that an underlying sleep complaint, if still present, can be evaluated without excessive contamination by multiple drug use.

Rebound insomnia and anxiety may appear shortly following the withdrawal of benzodiazepine medication that has been regularly taken for a period of weeks to months. The shorter the half-life of the compound, the sooner rebound symptoms will appear after the drug is stopped. Thus triazolam (Halcion), with a half-life of several hours, may be associated with rebound insomnia the first night it is not taken following days to 2 weeks of nightly administration. Some patients who have regularly taken benzodiazepine hypnotics with very short half-lives experience early morning awakening that has been attributed to an intranight drug withdrawal-type phenomenon. Temazepam (Restoril), with a half-life of about 10 hours, may have rebound symptoms delayed for a day or two, whereas very long-acting compounds, such as flurazepam (Dalmane) and diazepam (Valium), with half-lives of up to 100 hours, may have rebound insomnia and anxiety appear up to 1–2 weeks following drug termination. In such cases it is important to ascertain whether a true rebound phenomenon is occurring or whether the symptoms represent reemergence of the original symptoms for which the medications may have been prescribed in the first place. Rebound symptoms will subside, whereas reemergence of the primary pathology likely will not. Benzodiazepine withdrawal symptoms might include symptoms such as *muscle twitching*, *tinnitus*, *paresthesias*, and *visual disturbances*, which are uncommon in a generalized anxiety disorder (3).

Differential diagnosis of drug-related insomnias must also consider the possibility of more than one cause of insomnia being present simultaneously. Additionally, in the case of insomnias considered to be side effects of drugs administered for other reasons, should those drugs be reduced in order to ameliorate the insomnia, other underlying psychiatric or physiological conditions may reemerge that may also disrupt sleep. When looking for coexisting diagnoses in the patient who has been abusing drugs, it is important to be aware that symptoms of depression and anxiety or panic are frequent during the first 2 weeks after drug withdrawal; a formal diagnosis of depression or anxiety should be deferred until this period has passed. Evaluation for the use of tricyclic antidepressants to treat such depression should wait until at least 10–14 days after withdrawal. Symptoms such as hypomania that occur during the protracted withdrawal state, i.e., much longer than 2 weeks, offer even greater diagnostic confusion, but they should generally be treated as one would treat them in the nondrug-dependent patient. A PSG may be necessary to clarify diagnosis after sedative withdrawal.

TREATMENT

Insomnia related to severe substance abuse should be treated with rapid inpatient detoxification, appropriate medical management of withdrawal symptoms, and group, individual, and family supportive treatments as necessary.

Drug dependency insomnias must eventually be treated by withdrawal of the offending agent. Withdrawal must be slow—no more than one therapeutic dose per week—and the patient should be cautioned about the insomnia that likely will ensue. We generally prefer that such long-lasting and persistent insomnias be managed behaviorally to the fullest extent possible, with support from the physician, from emphasis on sleep hygiene, and from self-control and sleep restriction techniques, as outlined in a later section of this chapter. The use of L-tryptophan 1–5 g hs may be beneficial for both the substance abuse patient and the sedative-hypnotic-dependent patient during and shortly after the withdrawal period. Many patients will complain of chronic fatigue secondary to the protracted insomnia that will accompany and follow withdrawal. It is possible that a state of catecholamine depletion may accompany withdrawal, which may cause an independent insomnia. Such patients may benefit from the use of a sedating antidepressant such as doxepin, nortriptyline, trimipramine, or amitriptyline. These drugs should be started in low doses, e.g., 25–50 mg hs, and gradually increased until a sedative effect is achieved. The patient should be closely monitored and tapered off the antidepressant medication as soon as a significant period of stability ensues.

Some alcohol-dependent patients have started out with a glass of wine or a drink at bedtime to help them sleep, and have gradually escalated their alcohol usage to significant proportions, although still using it just once a day at bedtime. This group is often best managed by replacing the alcohol with an effective dose of a benzodiazepine hs and then gradually reducing this by one therapeutic equivalent per week as described above for sedative-hypnotic withdrawal.

Rebound insomnia and anxiety are best handled by advising the patient of their possible occurrence, and then withdrawing the medication very slowly in small dosage increments. Again, it is important with the longer half-life agents to differentiate between rebound symptoms and reemergence of the original symptoms, which may need additional specific treatment. Advising the patient ahead of time can be important, for if the symptoms are seen as a "normal" and expected phenomenon, they have a less ominous implication and may be better handled.

It is important to remember that during the treatment of drug dependency-related insomnias another form of sleep disorder may be unmasked. Therefore, it is important to go back through the differential diagnosis of the sleep disorders in such cases, and consider a PSG if necessary to clarify the previously masked diagnosis.

■ CIRCADIAN RHYTHM-BASED SLEEP DISORDERS

We consider here two general groupings of circadian rhythm-based sleep disorders. The first group includes disorders characterized by a persistent inability to entrain the circadian rhythm of the sleep cycle to that of the rest of the world. These disorders include delayed sleep phase syndrome, advanced sleep phase syndrome, non-24-hour sleep-wake cycle, and irregular sleep-wake cycle. The second group consists of disorders manifested in persons who are struggling to readjust their circadian function to new situations imposed by workshift change or by travel across time zones, including shift work sleep disorder and jet lag.

DELAYED SLEEP PHASE SYNDROME

PRESENTING COMPLAINTS

- Sleep onset insomnia, with difficulty falling asleep until very late at night or early in the morning
- Difficulty awakening in the early morning
- Daytime grogginess and fatigue, especially on days requiring early rising
- Feeling of being alert and energetic late in the evening
- Occasional complaints of depression, especially in adolescents

CLINICAL PRESENTATION

The typical patient with delayed sleep phase syndrome may be up until dawn trying to fall asleep. Once asleep, the patient will have normal quality sleep, which will last a normal time, unless interrupted by the alarm clock or by another external disturbance (4). The patient may feel well rested on days following a normal sleep period but be sleepy or groggy on days requiring early arising. These patients often become more awake and alert as the day progresses, and frequently enjoy working late into the night, when others are tired and ready to go to bed. They are often characterized as "night owls." Most adult patients show little sign of anxiety or mood disturbance other than frustration over long sleep latency.

INCIDENCE

It has been estimated that as many as 10% of the cases of chronic insomnia may be attributable to delayed sleep phase syndrome. Many individuals with this syndrome may adjust work and activity patterns around their circadian-induced sleep problem and never seek treatment.

In children, delayed sleep phase syndrome may rank as among the more common causes of sleep disturbances ("I don't want to go to bed—I'm not tired," followed by "I can't get up—I'm too tired"). (For discussion of this syndrome in children, see Chapter 8.)

ETIOLOGY AND PATHOPHYSIOLOGY

The physiological and sleep pattern correlates of circadian rhythms have been discussed previously in Chapter 2. Persons with delayed sleep phase syndrome may lack the ability to entrain their circadian rhythms to a period less than 24 hours. Once they have delayed their sleep-wake rhythms, such individuals are, therefore, unable to advance the rhythm to allow an earlier sleeping period.

The basic period of circadian rhythms, and possibly their entrainability, may be heritable traits. In families where one parent has delayed sleep phase syndrome, one or more children will also frequently demonstrate a similar sleep tendency.

LABORATORY FINDINGS

Laboratory studies are usually not necessary or particularly helpful in evaluation and treatment of delayed sleep phase syndrome. When these patients are studied in the sleep laboratory, they show prolonged sleep latency, followed by polysomnographically normal sleep, with delayed awakening until the sleep need has been met.

DIFFERENTIAL DIAGNOSIS

It is usually possible to make the diagnosis on the basis of history. A sleep diary kept for a 2-week period can be of considerable help. Patients will typically sleep unusually late on weekends or holidays, attempting to recoup the sleep lost during the week, when they have to arise early. A record of daytime sleepiness will usually show a progressive increase in daytime sleepiness as the week progresses.

The most common mimic of delayed sleep phase syndrome is *poor sleep hygiene*, with an intraweek circadian desynchronization. Many people have a morning arising time during their work week that is much earlier than that of the weekend. Because of the sleep rhythm's ease in adapting to phase delay, it is easy to sleep until 10:00 A.M. or even later on weekends. The person who sleeps very late on Sunday morning will not have his or her normal urge to fall asleep until 2:00 to 3:00 A.M. early the next morning. This shift in arising time on Sunday morning will typically result in sleep onset insomnia on Sunday night as well as on other days early in the week, with secondary tiredness and the tendency to oversleep on Monday morning. Establishing a rigorous morning arising time, including weekends, for a period of 2–3 weeks will usually clear up this problem. If this schedule fails to help, one must then be suspicious of delayed sleep phase syndrome.

Sometimes somewhat *socially isolated* (perhaps mildly schizoid) or *socially anxious* individuals seem to develop delayed sleep phase symptoms as a way to keep social conflicts and/or contacts to a minimum during waking hours. In these patients, the sleep pattern develops as a psychological defense, and this must be considered in setting up a treatment program.

It is important to closely screen for *affective and anxiety disorders* to make sure that the morning difficulty in arising is not an aspect of a tendency for mood to be worse in the morning in depression, or a means to avoid morning family interactions that produce anxiety.

Adolescents with delayed sleep phase syndrome frequently have problems with depression, loneliness, isolation, poor family and peer relationships, and poor school performance. Many of their problems may resolve with appropriate treatment of the phase delay.

TREATMENT

The treatment for the intraweek circadian desynchronization problem is good sleep hygiene—the strict adherence to keeping arising times constant 7 days per week, with no more than 1 hour variability from weekdays to weekends.

It is usually advisable to initially try good sleep hygiene even in those individuals suspected to have a true delayed sleep phase syndrome. It is the easiest treatment form to implement and to adhere to, and some cases do resolve. If the implementation of good sleep hygiene is ineffective, several other treatments are available:

1. *Chronotherapy* consists of placing the patient on a 27-hour day, progressively phase-delaying the sleep cycle about 3 hours each sleep-wake period until sleep onset time has been moved essentially around the clock to the time the patient considers the appropriate bedtime. Each sleep period must be strictly limited to 7 or 8 hours maximum, with no napping allowed. This treatment is frequently effective, so long as a rigorous morning arising time is maintained following the completion of the phase-delay portion of the treatment so that the sleep-wake rhythm does not have an opportunity to continue to phase-delay. Staying up unusually late (e.g., for a party) may once again lead to a desynchronization. The disadvantages of this treatment method are primarily the disturbance in daily schedule required to complete the phase delay. For several days the patient will have to sleep through the day uninterrupted, and appropriate arrangements must be made for time off the job, child care, etc. Some patients will have to repeat the treatment at intervals to keep rhythms synchronized.
2. An *alternative method of chronotherapy* is to keep the patient up all night one night and then attempt to phase-advance 90 minutes beginning the next evening. This procedure can be repeated each weekend to reinforce phase advance without the weekday disruption caused by the typical 5- to 7-day course of chronotherapy.
3. *Bright light exposure* immediately after awakening (2,500 lux

for 1–2 hours) has been found to advance sleep onset effectively, and may successfully treat delayed sleep phase syndrome. Further refinement of this technique, especially regarding duration and timing of light exposure, may result in bright light exposure eventually heading the list of recommended treatments because of its safety and lack of disruption of daytime activities. Bright light exposure may also be useful to keep circadian rhythms synchronized once established (5).

4. *Antidepressant medications*, including lithium, tricyclics, monoamine oxidase inhibitors, and second-generation tricyclics, all appear to facilitate the entrainment of circadian rhythms. At present, these medications would not appear to be the treatment of choice for uncomplicated delayed sleep phase syndrome, because we do not yet know enough about mechanisms of action and indications. However, we have seen a number of cases of delayed sleep phase syndrome complicated with affective disorder that have responded well to antidepressant medication, and would consider pharmacotherapy as an appropriate therapeutic consideration for the patient who does not respond to chronotherapy.

ADVANCED SLEEP PHASE SYNDROME

Much rarer than delayed sleep phase syndrome is the advanced sleep phase syndrome. The typical patient will complain of falling asleep at 8:00 or earlier in the evening and waking up between 3:00 and 5:00 in the morning. The origin of this syndrome is not yet clear. Differential diagnosis includes (a) *affective disorders*, which are often associated with an apparent advance of aspects of sleep rhythms, and (b) a *habit pattern* of early bedtime to avoid evening social interactions or responsibilities.

TREATMENT

1. If there is evidence of significant depression, consider the use of a nonsedating antidepressant such as desipramine. The administration of this medication can be coupled with a suggestion that the patient very slowly attempt to delay evening bedtime by 15 minutes every several days.

2. If there is no evidence of affective disorder, and if the suggestion of very slowly delaying the sleep period 15 minutes at a time is ineffective, consider bright light therapy or chronotherapy.
3. Bright light therapy for advanced sleep phase syndrome should consist of 1–2 hours exposure (2,500 lux) in the evening between 7:00 and 9:00 P.M.
4. There have been case reports of the effectiveness of chronotherapy, with the patient going to bed 3 hours earlier each night until the sleep cycle is phase-advanced back to a normal bedtime.

NON-24-HOUR SLEEP-WAKE CYCLE

This is a rare condition in which the length of the sleep-wake cycle can become much longer than the typical 24 hours. Some people have been known to develop 30- to 50-hour cycles with prolonged wake times followed by longer-than-normal sleep. This syndrome is most often seen in those who are blind.

DIFFERENTIAL DIAGNOSIS

Frequent stimulant abuse would appear to be the most frequent mimic of this syndrome. It is important to obtain an adequate drug history as well as to have the patient very carefully graph out the periodicity of the sleeping and waking. Lengthened but severely erratic sleep periods can be an aspect of a schizoid avoidance of social contact, as well as a symptom of sporadic hypnotic and alcohol abuse.

TREATMENT

There is no effective treatment yet known for the true, prolonged non-24-hour sleep-wake cycle, although appropriately timed bright light treatment might be considered. Even some blind individuals will respond to light if the retinal-hypothalamic tracts are intact. Marginal cases may respond to the protocol for delayed sleep phase syndrome. Any evidence of drug abuse, personality disorder, or affective disorder should be treated appropriately.

IRREGULAR SLEEP-WAKE CYCLE

Normal circadian function can be virtually abolished in a number of illnesses, including severe dementia, head injury, recovery from coma, recovery from drug and alcohol intoxication, and severe depression, as well as in those cases of persistent CNS stimulant, CNS depressant, or hypnotic dependency. Some mentally retarded or otherwise brain-damaged persons may exhibit an irregular sleep-wake cycle.

TREATMENT

Treatment should be based on appropriately treating the underlying condition and then reinforcing regularity of the sleep-wake cycle with normal daytime activity, regular exercise, meals, and attention to good sleep hygiene. Regular bright white-light treatment would perhaps be worth a trial.

SHIFT WORK SLEEP DISORDER

PRESENTING COMPLAINTS

Presenting complaints (occurring in a shift worker) include the following:

- Chronic fatigue, drowsiness, and impaired work performance
- Difficulty initiating sleep
- Decreased duration and poor quality of sleep
- Complaints of job stress, depression, emotional problems, and family life disruption
- Somatic complaints, especially related to the gastrointestinal system (such as gastritis and constipation)
- Increased use of alcohol, tranquilizers, or sleeping pills to decrease stress and increase sleep
- Excessive smoking and caffeine consumption to aid alertness

CLINICAL PRESENTATION

The shift worker's most common complaint is disrupted sleep, with difficulty initiating and maintaining sleep, and poor sleep quality. These patients also experience chronic fatigue, drowsiness, and dozing off at work in association with the disrupted sleep. They have an increased number of accidents and attention-related mistakes. Shift workers are also reported to have a higher incidence of chronic depression, emotional problems, family life dysfunction, excessive drug (including cigarettes) and alcohol use, ulcers, and elevated cardiovascular risk.

Whereas some shift workers will seek help from physicians or employers, others have problems that only come to light after on-the-job accidents, falling asleep at work, detection of drug or alcohol use, or by workers quitting to avoid shifting (6, 7). Shift workers' sleep and related symptoms have been called *shift workers' sleep disorder* or *shift work maladaptation syndrome*.

INCIDENCE

It is estimated that in 1980 26% of male workers and 18% of female workers had jobs that required shift rotation. Epidemiological studies have suggested that about 25% of shift workers (or 6% of the American work force) may be suffering from some aspect of a shift work maladaptation syndrome (7).

ETIOLOGY AND PATHOPHYSIOLOGY

Shift work sleep disorder or maladaptation syndrome has been postulated to be due to either (a) disturbances in regulation of circadian rhythms secondary to work shift time changes, or (b) sleep loss, or possibly both.

A sudden work shift change of 8 hours leaves the sleep-wake schedule suddenly out of synchronization with other circadian biorhythms. With circadian physiology in desynchrony, sleep can be difficult to initiate, less restful when obtained, and more often interrupted and shortened in length. Being forced to function out of synchrony appears to "flatten" circadian biorhythms, with less variation in body temperature throughout the day. This flattening may cause additional problems over time, possibly contributing to a chronic inability to sustain normal sleep.

It has also been postulated that the sleep loss itself, and perhaps the means used to combat it (alcohol, sedatives) and reinforce alertness (stimulants, cigarettes, food), are a major cause of shift workers' symptoms.

Another major and related factor in the etiology of shift

work disorders is the disruption of family life by frequent absence, tiredness or depression, and the need to sleep during daytime hours.

LABORATORY STUDIES

A PSG would typically demonstrate increased sleep latency, numerous arousals during sleep, and early awakening, as well as sleep efficiency below 85%. A PSG, however, is usually not needed unless there is a suspicion of an additional primary sleep disorder.

DIFFERENTIAL DIAGNOSIS

Because of the high incidence of emotional problems within the shift worker group, the patient should be evaluated for affective and anxiety disorders, requiring psychotherapy or medication, in addition to a careful medical and sleep history. A history of returning to a normal sleep pattern during vacations or time off rotation can help with diagnosis.

One should look carefully for evidence of alcoholism or drug dependency, insomnia due to poor sleep hygiene such as excessive caffeine and cigarette use, or use of alcohol as a regular sedative. Many workers aggravate their condition with poor sleep hygiene, which complicates diagnosis and treatment.

TREATMENT

The body's ability to adapt to shift changes is in part a function of the direction of the shift, which determines whether a phase delay (easier to adapt to) or a phase advance (harder to adapt to) is required. An 8-hour shift change that allows sleep time to shift 8 hours later (phase delay) can be adapted to in about 3 days. If the sleep time has to shift 8 hours earlier (phase advance), it may take 6–7 days to adapt. For workers with no regular shifts but constant "on call" schedules, there may never be a chance to develop adequate synchrony.

Two general approaches to treatment include (a) treatment of the patient, and (b) attempts to encourage the workplace to adapt to workers' needs.

SHIFT WORKER RECOMMENDATIONS

1. Attempt to maintain a *regular sleep and meal schedule* whenever possible.
2. *Encourage naps* to limit sleep loss.
3. Practice *good sleep hygiene*, especially reducing alcohol and caffeine consumption. If sleeping during daylight hours, ensure adequate darkness and screening from noise and interruption as much as possible.
4. Some patients will benefit from *short-half-life hypnotics* to aid in initiating sleep, but this benefit must be weighed against potential decrease in daytime alertness. The development of dependency must be discouraged.

ORGANIZATIONAL RECOMMENDATIONS

1. Benefits in worker satisfaction, productivity, and health have been shown when workers are allowed to change shifts in a *phase-delayed direction* (i.e., night shift to day shift) (8).
2. *Napping should be encouraged* at times as a way to aid in maintaining alertness on long work stints.
3. *Avoid excessively long shifts* whenever possible.
4. Current research on *bright light exposure* offers some real promise for the future as a means of resetting circadian rhythms more quickly. This research may have implications for the workplace, but it is probably too early to recommend a specific implementation at this time.
5. A work-scheduling system called the "*European twos*" seems to be favored by workers over other longer-period work shift schedules (e.g., 1 week on each shift). In this system the workers spend 2 days on each shift consecutively and then have 3 days off. Although circadian rhythms are maximally disrupted during the 2 days on night shift, workers can quickly return to their typical routine, and some claim to get more sleep with this system.

JET LAG

Jet lag is a travel-induced circadian rhythm desynchronization, with sleep-wake and other circadian physiological rhythms suddenly being out of synchrony with the new 24-hour light-dark cycle. The body can adapt easily to a time change of about an hour a day; thus there was no jet lag-like condition in times of slower travel, when it was rare that a time zone (about 800 miles in midcontinent latitudes) was crossed in less than a day. As travel speeded up, and as time zones were crossed more rapidly, jet lag became a problem.

Symptoms of jet lag include difficulty sleeping at the new sleep time, daytime sleepiness and fatigue, and impaired performance during the new daylight hours. The body's 24-hour rhythms, such as those for serum cortisol and body temperature, remain on the old time, and shift slowly to the new time, requiring about 1 day to adapt for each hour of time change. Jet lag symptoms are usually more pronounced for travel west to east (which entails a phase advance), and less pronounced for travel east to west (which entails a phase delay). Thus travelers flying from the United States to Europe have more difficulty than when flying from Europe to the United States.

TREATMENT

Treatment of jet lag includes both behavioral and pharmacological components. It is helpful, if possible, to lead the time change by beginning to shift sleep and activity patterns ahead of time. In any case, it is best to change to the new rest activity schedule immediately upon arrival, and sleep at the new sleep time, eat at the new meal times, and work at the new work time.

Certain special diets have been recommended to decrease jet lag symptoms, but none has yet been empirically demonstrated to significantly improve speed of adaptation. Treatment also appropriately includes a short-half-life benzodiazepine hypnotic (e.g., triazolam 0.125 or 0.25 mg or temazepam 15–30 mg) for several nights at the new sleep time. Long-half-life benzodiazepines should be avoided. It is possible that early morning bright white-light exposure, such as an hour's walk outside in the daylight at the new time zone, will help more quickly reentrain the body's circadian physiology.

■ PERIODIC LIMB MOVEMENTS (NOCTURNAL MYOCLONUS) AND RESTLESS LEG SYNDROME

PRESENTING COMPLAINTS OF PERIODIC LIMB MOVEMENTS OF SLEEP (NOCTURNAL MYOCLONUS)

- Patient usually complains primarily of chronic insomnia, either frequent awakenings or difficulty falling asleep
- Patient may complain of leg jerking
- Bed partner complains that the patient kicks during sleep
- Bedclothes frequently in disarray in the morning
- Patient may have associated restless leg symptoms
- Complaints aggravated by tricyclics or dopa
- PLMS may present as EDS

PRESENTING COMPLAINTS OF RESTLESS LEG SYNDROME

- Uncomfortable "crawling" feelings, usually in the calf of the leg, that begin when the patient lies down to sleep
- Crawling feelings relieved by movement (e.g., walking)

CLINICAL PRESENTATION

Periodic limb movements of sleep (nocturnal myoclonus) and restless leg syndrome are considered together, for they frequently occur together and they may share certain features. While these conditions were originally called nocturnal myoclonus, more recent terms include periodic leg movements of sleep (PLMS), periodic limb movements of sleep (also PLMS), and periodic movements during sleep (PMS), all of which do not account for the fact that the movements may occur during wakefulness. Although these terms will all be found in common usage today, we will generally use periodic limb movements of sleep (PLMS) in this chapter when referring to the syndrome.

PLMS consist of periodic (every 20 to 40 seconds) contractions of the tibialis anterior with dorsiflexion of the ankle and toes, resulting in a leg jerk, or a slight kick, frequently accompanied by a short EEG arousal. The bed partner may complain that the patient is very restless, or that he or she kicks for prolonged periods during the night. The patient usually is not aware of the leg jerks but only of the sense of being awake or waking frequently. PLMS may also be seen when the patient naps in a chair during the day.

Restless leg syndrome is a dysesthesia characterized by uncomfortable "creepy-crawly" sensations and/or prickly feelings in the calves of the legs that occur when the patient lies down to rest or sleep, and can be alleviated only by getting up and "walking them out" (9). Thus restless legs may not be a true sleep disorder, because the symptoms appear during wakefulness, but it certainly does interfere with sleep, and the patient frequently presents with a complaint of sleep onset insomnia. The patient may find it difficult to express the nature of the uncomfortable feelings in his or her legs, using at times somewhat strange terms such as a sense of "worms crawling," and the like.

PLMS may present as EDS, especially if nocturnal sleep is severely fragmented by the leg jerks.

INCIDENCE

An analysis of 5,000 patient records from 11 Sleep Disorders Centers reported by Coleman et al. (10) found that of the patients with DIMS, 12% had PLMS or restless leg syndrome as a cause. Normally sleeping subjects may exhibit PLMS but may not complain of insomnia. The incidence of PLMS is higher in males and increases with age, with some studies suggesting that up to 49% of subjects 65 and older have PLMS indices (number of limb jerks per hour of sleep) of 5 or greater (11). The incidence of PLMS is also higher in patients with narcolepsy or sleep apnea. Recent findings from our laboratory (12) suggest that PLMS may be relatively common even in chronic insomniac patients who have been prescreened by history for PLMS.

Restless leg syndrome has variously been estimated to be related to up to 10% of the cases of chronic insomnia, especially in older patients with medical disorders, in whom the syndrome is more common.

ETIOLOGY AND PATHOPHYSIOLOGY

In some cases PLMS and restless leg syndrome are apparently transmitted as an autosomal dominant with onset in the second decade and lifelong persistence. Both syndromes have been associated with a variety of medical disorders, including peripheral neuropathies, anemia, uremia, and chronic pulmonary disease. Restless leg syndrome per se has been linked to vitamin and mineral deficiencies, uremia, and malignancy, and recently has been estimated to occur in up to 30% of patients with rheumatoid arthritis (13). A familial syndrome of nocturnal painful cramping and leg jerking has also been described (14). Syndromes similar to PLMS and restless leg syndrome also accompany Huntington's chorea and amyotrophic lateral sclerosis. PLMS may also be associated with a "fibrositis syndrome" termed rheumatic pain modulation disorder, with an accompanying nonrestorative alpha-delta-like sleep pattern. This disorder has a higher incidence in women.

The pathophysiology of PLMS is unclear. This syndrome is not accompanied by abnormal EEG activity, nor does it appear to presage the onset of other motor or neurological symptoms. Recent studies suggest that PLMS are usually associated with a K complex and are accompanied by transient increases in heart rate, blood pressure, and a deepening of breathing, and thus may represent part of a complex arousal-like activity pattern (15). PLMS may also be associated with changes in sleep positions, and with the termination of breathing irregularities (e.g., short hypopneas or apneas) during sleep.

PLMS, with dorsiflexion of the ankle and toes, and sometimes fanning, are similar to the Babinski reflex: These movements are sometimes accompanied by changes in autonomic activity and EEG suggestive of an origin similar to, if not the same as, that of the Babinski reflex. The Babinski reflex elicited during wakefulness is indicative of pyramidal tract disease, but it can normally be elicited during non-REM sleep because of suppression of inhibitory suprasegmental influences during these sleep stages. Some evidence exists for increased segmental excitability of brain stem and spinal reflexes in patients with PLMS, which would implicate a mechanism(s) at the pontine (or more rostral) level (16).

LABORATORY FINDINGS

To be scored as a periodic limb movement, the tibialis anterior EMG should demonstrate bursts of activity of at least 0.5 seconds, but not more than 5.0 seconds, in duration. At least two such EMG bursts must occur within a 4- to 90-second interval (usually 20–40 seconds) for a leg jerk to be counted. The total number of leg jerks occurring during sleep is divided by the number of hours of sleep to provide a "myoclonic index" or "PLMS index." Myoclonic activity typically occurs in bouts during the night. Thus, for example, a bout of 30–60 or more PLMS may be followed by a period of one or more hours of fairly normal sleep, only to be followed again by another bout of PLMS. These movements can vary significantly from night to night, complicating assessment by sleep laboratory studies. Most patients with restless leg syndrome also demonstrate PLMS on a PSG, but not all patients demonstrating PLMS complain of restless legs.

The PLMS index must be interpreted in the context of other clinical and polysomnographic findings. It would seem that PLMS accompanied by evidence of arousal (alpha activity in the EEG, increase in chin muscle activity in the EMG) are of more concern than episodes showing no arousal; polysomnographic records should be scored and interpreted accordingly, with leg jerks associated with arousals separated from those not associated with arousals. Examples of PLMS without and with arousal are illustrated in Figures 3-2 and 3-3, respectively.

In our laboratory, we use the rule of thumb that a PLMS index of 12 or greater, with 50% or more of PLMS accompanied by evidence of EEG arousals, should be considered a potentially significant contributor to a complaint of insomnia and should merit treatment evaluation. There may be patients in whom lower indexes are of significance. The necessary research more specifically linking PLMS to insomnia has yet to be reported.

DIFFERENTIAL DIAGNOSIS

Restless leg syndrome is diagnosed by history. Suspicion of PLMS can also be raised by the history, but a PSG is required for definitive diagnosis. Patients treated for chronic insomnia, with-

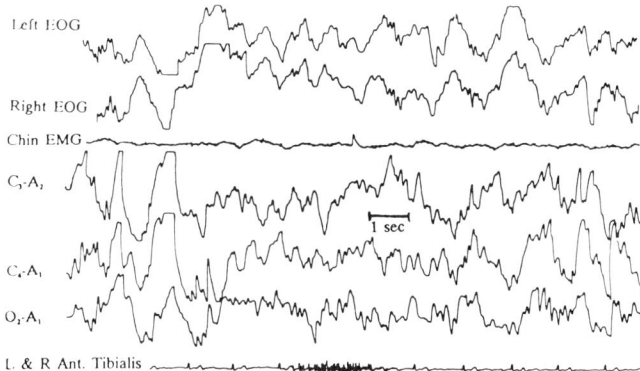

FIGURE 3-2. Polysomnogram showing a periodic limb movement that is not accompanied by arousal.
Leg jerk indicated by EMG burst in left and right leg (combined) tibialis anterior EMG (bottom channel). Ongoing Stage 3 sleep is not disrupted (no arousal).

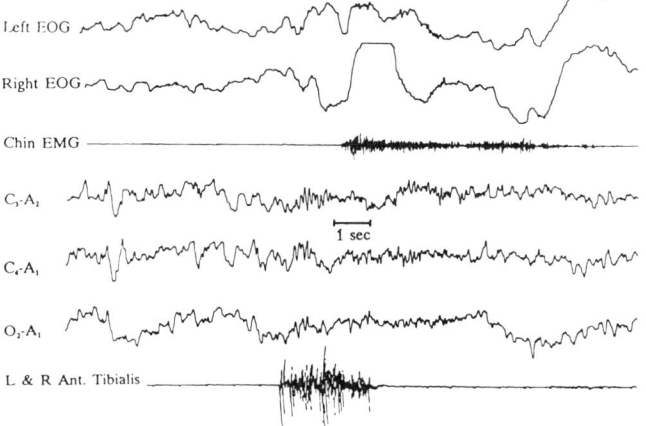

FIGURE 3-3. Polysomnogram showing a periodic limb movement that is accompanied by arousal.
Leg jerk in tibialis anterior EMG (bottom channel) is followed by EEG arousal, with increased chin muscle activity (EMG) and eye movement.

out benefit of a PSG, may have PLMS but remain undiagnosed. Thus this diagnosis should be suspected in patients not responding to other insomnia treatments.

Specific conditions to consider in the differential diagnosis of PLMS include:

- *Hypnic jerks*. These sudden body jerks often occur at sleep onset and are frequently accompanied by imagery such as missing a step. These sleep-onset phenomena, also called "sleep starts," are similar to a startle reaction and are considered to be normal phenomena.
- *Nocturnal leg cramps* in the calves and in the muscles of the sole of the foot—"charlie horses"—usually relieved by stretching. Occasionally, nocturnal severe cramps may also respond to quinine, a low dose of codeine, or benadryl. There may be familial versions of this disorder that, if frequent, may respond to clonazepam 0.25 mg hs.
- *Peripheral vascular insufficiency* that may have associated nocturnal leg cramps. An evaluation for arteriosclerotic disease might be indicated.
- *Peripheral neuropathy* with associated burning pain and discomfort.
- *Other myoclonic-like activities* associated with CNS degenerative conditions, which should be apparent upon physical examination.
- The "*painful legs and moving toes*" syndrome—a rare syndrome that includes pain in the feet with spontaneous movement of the toes (17).
- *Epileptic myoclonus*, which is usually associated with EEG abnormalities.
- *Nocturnal cataclysms* (18), which are frightening nocturnal episodes that have reportedly accompanied clomipramine use. These episodes have been relieved by clonazepam.
- *Episodic fragmentary myoclonus*—a rare disorder seen predominantly in males, characterized by brief (<150 milliseconds), random, multifocal, asynchronous muscle jerks occurring predominantly during non-REM sleep, with a clinical complaint of either insomnia or EDS (19).

Perhaps the major problem in clinical assessment of PLMS

is to decide to what degree the disorder contributes to the overall sleep complaint. Nocturnal myoclonus as an isolated finding in the absence of sleep complaints is called "essential nocturnal myoclonus." When insomnia is the complaint, however, clinical skills must be utilized to estimate to what extent PLMS contributes to the sleep complaint, and whether other causes for the sleep complaint may coexist, such as a psychophysiological or learned insomnia or a concurrent psychiatric disorder. Treatment for more than one disorder may be necessary.

TREATMENT

The treatment of PLMS and restless leg syndrome is complicated by the fact that we do not understand the pathophysiology of these disorders, and therefore a rational treatment cannot yet be advanced. It is also possible that PLMS represents a group of disorders with common symptoms but differing etiologies and pathophysiologies; only further research will clarify this possibility. All pharmacological treatments appear symptomatic, and it is not yet known how long they might be effective, or if they modify the underlying PLMS syndrome. PLMS (or nocturnal myoclonus) has been reported to respond to the following treatments:

CLONAZEPAM AND TEMAZEPAM

Clonazepam (Clonopin) 1.0 mg hs and temazepam (Restoril) 30 mg hs (20) have been used for treatment of PLMS. In both cases it appears the frequency of leg jerks is not decreased, but patients are better able to sleep through them. The long-term use of these agents for PLMS should be approached with caution and might best be handled with an intermittent treatment regimen including substantial drug-free intervals.

BACLOFEN

Baclofen 20 to 40 mg hs has been shown to decrease PLMS-induced sleep fragmentation and improve subjective sleep quality. The drug increased PLMS frequency, however; thus its role in the treatment of PLMS is unclear (21). Baclofen is a GABA (gamma-aminobutyric acid) II mimetic and may work by reducing excitatory transmitter release at the spinal level, resulting in hyperpolarization of afferent terminals.

CODEINE

Codeine 30 to 60 mg hs and other opioid compounds have been reported in uncontrolled studies to (a) decrease the frequency of PLMS and to result in subjective sleep improvement, and (b) decrease the complaint of restless leg syndrome as well (22). The long-term use of opioid compounds should be considered with caution as with other sedative-hypnotic agents.

BIOFEEDBACK

Biofeedback aimed at increasing skin temperature of the foot has recently been reported to diminish sleep complaints in PLMS patients who complain of cold feet. This option, if available, might be considered for selected patients (23).

OTHER TREATMENT STRATEGIES

The treatment of PLMS occurring in the presence of other disorders, such as sleep-related breathing disorders, narcolepsy, or sleep complaints related to affective disorders, is complicated by the fact that *tricyclics*, frequently used in the treatment of these disorders, *may substantially aggravate PLMS*. Lithium has also been reported to aggravate PLMS.

Restless leg syndrome has been reported in uncontrolled studies to respond variably to iron supplements (if anemia is present); trace minerals; L-tryptophan; opiates, including codeine at doses as low as 10 mg hs; propoxyphene; methadone hydrochloride 5–20 mg; oxycodone 5–15 mg; dopamine agonists, including L-dopa 200 mg (with the peripheral decarboxylase inhibitor benserazide) and bromocriptine 2.5–5.0 mg; benzodiazepines such as diazepam or clonazepam; and baclofen. The multiplicity of proposed treatments and lack of controlled studies of effectiveness suggest that treatment strategy might best begin with the most innocuous agent and proceed to more active compounds only if required, attending (and alerting patients) to possible side effects and drug complications.

Studies in an animal model of restless leg syndrome suggest that certain benzodiazepines (clonazepam and flunitrazepam) are much more effective than others (e.g., diazepam) in relieving leg jerks. It is not known if this difference is clinically relevant.

■ SLEEP APNEA INSOMNIA

PRESENTING COMPLAINTS

- Insomnia, with sleep disruption and frequent awakenings
- Possible complaints of depression and/or decreased libido
- Occasional complaints of difficulty getting a breath, or gasping
- Occasional complaint of snoring

CLINICAL PRESENTATION

Patients exhibiting frequent central apneas during sleep often present with a complaint of insomnia, and occasionally also snoring, depression, and decreased libido. They usually do not have EDS or other manifestations typical of the obstructive apnea syndrome. Patients most often have no direct respiratory complaint, although occasionally they have a sense of momentary breathlessness, or they experience difficulty getting a breath, or gasping respiration (not true shortness of breath). The bed partner will frequently give a history of repeated short pauses in the patient's respiration during sleep.

INCIDENCE

Studies of the presence of significant central apnea in adult insomniac populations have ranged from 1 to 12%; our experience is compatible with the lower end of this range. While central apnea is probably among the rarer causes of chronic insomnia in younger patients, its incidence increases with advancing age, as does the incidence of mixed and obstructive apneas (24).

Central apneas occurring alone are relatively uncommon; more frequently they occur in combination with obstructive apneas, or as antecedents to obstructive events, in which case they are termed mixed apneas.

The incidence of central apnea is increased at higher elevations, and sleep-related respiratory disturbances may account for many of the sleep complaints experienced by most individuals during the first several nights at high altitude (e.g., while camping, mountain climbing, or on a skiing vacation).

ETIOLOGY AND PATHOPHYSIOLOGY

Central apneas occur when the respiratory efforts of the diaphragm and intercostal muscles cease, and breathing is momentarily interrupted. The apneas are usually terminated by a brief arousal, thus producing the subjective sense of not sleeping and the complaint of insomnia. These apneas, as seen on an EEG, not infrequently occur at the transition point between wakefulness and Stage 1 sleep.

Respiration during sleep is closely related to the activity of chemoreceptors, including the carotid body for hypoxia and medullary chemosensors for hypercapnia. Individuals with abnormally functioning chemosensors (e.g., patients with Ondine's curse) may hypoventilate during the day and exhibit respiratory abnormalities during sleep, including both central and obstructive apneas. While hypoxia may increase breathing rate during sleep, it is thought that Pco_2 is a major factor in the maintenance of respiratory regularity during sleep. If Pco_2 decreases for whatever reason (e.g., hyperventilation secondary to hypoxia at high altitude), irregular or periodic breathing, and possibly central apnea, ensue. The sleep state itself appears to be associated with a depression in both hypoxic and hypercapnic ventilatory drives as well, which may account for the association between wake-sleep transitions and central apneas. The presence of central apnea does not necessarily imply a disorder of the chemosensors, because patients with substantial apnea may exhibit normally functioning chemosensors, as measured by current techniques (25).

The hemodynamic consequences of central apneas are not as profound as with obstructive or mixed apneas. Oxygen desaturations are relatively small, and relatively small increases in pulmonary artery pressure and systemic pressure have been described as accompanying central apneas.

Several medical disorders may be accompanied by central apneas, including congestive heart failure, diabetes mellitus, nasal obstruction (from either anatomic abnormalities or nasal congestion due to a common cold), and several neurological disorders, including familial dysautonomia, Shy-Drager syndrome, encephalitis, and brain stem tumors or infarctions.

LABORATORY FINDINGS

Central apneas are defined as loss of both respiratory effort and flow for a period of at least 10 seconds. (See Figure 4-3 for illustration of a polygraph tracing showing a central apnea.) Most central apneas tend to be short (<20 seconds) and have minimal hemodynamic consequences. A nocturnal PSG demonstrating a central apnea index of greater than 5 per hour in a patient complaining of chronic insomnia should be considered as evidence that the apneas could be contributing to the insomnia complaint. Apnea indices are sometimes considerably greater than 5, with several hundred apneas occurring during the night. In such cases the relation of the apnea to the insomnia complaint is clearer, and one is more comfortable attributing the insomnia to the apnea.

DIFFERENTIAL DIAGNOSIS

Insomnia based upon central apnea is essentially a sleep laboratory diagnosis. One's index of suspicion is heightened when patients complain of a sense of difficulty getting their breath, or of breathlessness upon waking. Snoring, or a bed partner's complaint that the patient breathes irregularly or stops breathing, should also raise the index of suspicion. Once the diagnosis of central sleep apnea is made on the basis of a PSG, it is important to evaluate the patient for treatable causes such as congestive heart failure, nasal obstruction, and other less common causes listed above. The more common sleep-related breathing disorders associated with EDS are discussed in Chapter 4.

More common perhaps is the situation in which a patient with other causes of insomnia has a minimally increased number of central apneas. In this situation, contributing factors such as anxiety, psychological factors, stress, and evidence of a psychophysiological insomnia come into play. In such cases it is important not to over-treat the apnea, or to initially place too much emphasis on central apnea as the major cause of the insomnia. Rather, the treatment strategy should emphasize efforts aimed at the other possible causative factors, as appropriate. Treatment should *not* include the use of sedative-hypnotic agents, which may aggravate the apnea component.

TREATMENT

Central apneas secondary to medical disorders should be approached by appropriate treatment of the medical disorder first. Treatment of central apnea per se is not entirely satisfactory. At higher elevations, *acetazolamide* (Diamox) 250 mg hs to + id may prove helpful. Acetazolamide is a carbonic anhydrase inhibitor that produces a mild metabolic acidosis and may shift the hypercapnic ventilatory response to the left. This agent has been shown to be helpful in improving breathing during sleep at high altitude, and perhaps in preventing other symptoms of altitude sickness as well. Its mechanism of action, aside from producing a metabolic acidosis, is unclear, but may include direct action as a respiratory stimulant. Acetazolamide may not work as well for central apnea-related symptoms at lower (<5,000 feet) elevations. It has also not been shown to be effective for prolonged periods. Some patients have developed obstructive apneas during acetazolamide treatment, suggesting that a follow-up PSG is indicated, especially if clinical improvement is less than adequate.

Clomipramine, a tricyclic, has been of occasional benefit both in treating central apnea and in reducing associated snoring complaints. However, its mechanism of action is unclear.

Oxygen administration (1–2 liters/minute) has been shown to be effective in some cases. This approach should be tried in a closely supervised trial in a sleep laboratory, because some patients show a prolongation of their apneic events with worsening of hypoxemia.

Mechanical ventilation or *diaphragmatic pacemakers* have been used in severe cases of central apneas, but only as a last resort in patients with severe disease.

■ PSYCHOPHYSIOLOGICAL INSOMNIA

PRESENTING COMPLAINTS

- Difficulty falling asleep or staying asleep—usually of long duration
- Sleep complaints often more prominent in home bedroom
- Sleep complaints frequently began at time of stress or with a transient insomnia, and may co-vary with stress

- Sleep may be normal on vacation or in less-familiar environments
- Patient may have a long-standing history of "fragile sleep"

CLINICAL PRESENTATION

The term *psychophysiological insomnia* or "learned insomnia" describes those patients (often those who have never been good sleepers) who typically develop a chronic insomnia following a period of stress and continue to experience this insomnia even after the stress remits. It is thought that some patients may condition themselves to not sleep, that is, they may "learn" the insomnia. Sleep complaints tend to be fixed over time, or they may co-vary with the degree of daytime stress. Patients often tend to be tense or "wired" individuals, suggesting that some individuals are more prone than others for the development of psychophysiological insomnia. Sleep onset insomnia does not always characterize this disorder. These patients can often fall asleep rather easily, but they then may have several hours of wakefulness later in the night.

The term "psychophysiological insomnia" is actually a misnomer, however, because there are as of yet no physiological or psychophysiological profiles or tests that are specific to or pathognomonic of this diagnosis.

INCIDENCE

Psychophysiological insomnia represents the largest single category of nonpsychiatric chronic insomnia. While its exact incidence in the population has not been determined, and likely varies as a function of age, health, occupation, socioeconomic status, and geography, several studies have estimated that over 20% of the adult population experience a bout of chronic insomnia at some time during their lives (26), and this diagnostic category can be expected to make up a large proportion of those cases. Thus psychophysiological insomnia represents a major public and personal health problem, accounting for substantial personal disability and impaired work performance.

ETIOLOGY AND PATHOPHYSIOLOGY

Three factors appear important in the development of chronic psychophysiological insomnia: (a) predisposition or vulnerability, (b) life stress events, and (c) learning. *Predisposition* refers to both a higher incidence of measures related to psychopathology and quite possibly a specific vulnerability of neurophysiological sleep-inducing and sleep-maintaining mechanisms. Studies have shown that chronic insomnia populations tend to exhibit scores in the direction of psychopathology on a variety of psychological tests such as the Minnesota Multiphasic Personality Inventory (MMPI), and a higher incidence of Axis I and II diagnoses in the DSM-III-R classification. Patients who have a substantial psychiatric contribution to their insomnia are considered separately in Chapter 6. Nonetheless, many patients in the psychophysiological insomnia category may also have psychological contributions, although perhaps not severe enough to result in a formal DSM-III-R diagnosis. Such a contribution may result in greater reactivity to stress, greater concern with issues related to control, and greater vulnerability to life events impacting upon sleep-inducing and sleep-maintaining systems.

It has been suggested that patients vulnerable to chronic insomnia may have a predisposition as well in the direction of higher activity levels of the reticular activating system, resulting in easier sleep fragmentation (i.e., easier arousability in the face of stimuli), or impaired activity in forebrain sleep-inducing and sleep-maintaining systems, and that such components may be familial in origin. To date, however, such speculation remains just that, and such imputed biological contributions have yet to be formally identified.

It has also been suggested that certain types of insomnia, especially those characterized by deficiencies in Stage 3 and Stage 4 sleep, may be associated with disturbances in body temperature regulation, such that the expected prominent decreases in body temperature seen during the first several hours of sleep, and accompanied by transitions into Stage 3 and Stage 4 slow wave sleep, are absent or impaired (27).

Life stress events appear to play a role in the development of chronic insomnia. Chronic insomniac patients tend to have a greater number of life stress events during the year their insomnia began, particularly events related to loss and ill health (28). What is not clear is whether these individuals, for whatever reason, are not as able to handle stressful life events as are noninsomniac persons.

Learning appears to be important in many, if not most, cases of psychophysiological insomnia. Patients are thought to in some respects "learn" to arouse in their normal sleep setting. Typically, a patient will experience a transient stress-related insomnia, and after a couple of nights of prolonged sleep latency and perceived difficulty sleeping, the patient begins to be concerned about going to bed for fear of not being able to get to sleep. The fear response itself is then accompanied by increased anxiety and possibly autonomic arousal, such that the process of going to bed becomes associated with a central state conducive to continued wakefulness and increased arousal. The more concerned the patient becomes about not sleeping, the greater the arousal, thus setting up a vicious circle.

LABORATORY STUDIES

Polysomnography is usually not necessary for the diagnosis of psychophysiological insomnia, other than to exclude other causes of insomnia.

Most patients with psychophysiological insomnia will exhibit a prolonged sleep latency (>30 minutes), frequent awakenings, low total sleep time (<6 hours) and low sleep efficiency ($<85\%$), as well as a shift to lighter sleep stages on a PSG. Some patients will have a mild tachycardia (80–90 beats per minute) during slow wave sleep, suggesting increased autonomic activity. However, no specific set of findings are pathognomonic of psychophysiological insomnia.

Some patients may have less trouble sleeping in the nonhome laboratory environment, resulting in more normal-appearing PSGs. Thus the presence of a relatively normal PSG in the laboratory does not exclude the possibility of real sleep difficulties in the patient's normal sleep environment. Sleep history is important in this regard.

DIFFERENTIAL DIAGNOSIS

It should first be established that the patient has a true insomnia and is not just a typical *short sleeper*. Short sleepers, while not common, do exist, and may get along fine on 4–5 hours of sleep a night. They do not complain of EDS or fatigue, and usually they have no sleep complaints. Their families, however, seeing the patient up until midnight and then out of bed again at 4:00 A.M., assume there is a sleep problem and convince him or her to seek professional help. Such individuals need no specific treatment, although an explanation is helpful for family members.

Similarly, it should be ascertained that a true insomnia is in fact present, and not just a subjective sleep disturbance due to poor sleep habits or an atypical or erratic sleep schedule. Shift workers, or those with very erratic sleep schedules for varying reasons (e.g., computer hackers who like to work at night), frequently complain of poor sleep, which can be traced to their irregular sleep schedule. The *shift work sleep disorder* is a more chronic syndrome that includes prominent sleep complaints (see above).

A complaint of insomnia without objective findings is occasionally encountered. Although such individuals often present with a history compatible with psychophysiological insomnia, when studied in the sleep laboratory (usually after failing to respond to treatment) their sleep is found to be normal. These individuals have normal MMPI profiles and no specific evidence of psychopathology, and the cause of their complaint often remains obscure. Some may have a true psychophysiological insomnia, but one that only appears in their normal sleep environment. Occasionally, these individuals benefit merely from finding that their sleep in the laboratory is in fact normal.

Psychophysiological insomnia as a cause of chronic insomnia should not be diagnosed until other medical causes have been excluded, including drug dependency, PLMS (nocturnal myoclonus), central sleep apnea, psychiatric causes, poor sleep habits, and circadian rhythm disorders.

The diagnosis may be complicated in cases in which a sleep disturbance is based upon multiple etiologies, or is accompanied by poor sleep habits. The addition of a psychophysiological insomnia-type overlay to other types of insomnia must also be considered.

Additional rarer causes of chronic insomnia need to be excluded, including *childhood onset insomnia* and *REM arousal insomnia* (see below), as well as the non-24-hour sleep-wake cycle (discussed earlier in this chapter).

TREATMENT

Treatment of psychophysiological insomnia includes both behavioral and pharmacological components. Behavioral components include improved sleep hygiene, self-control techniques, and elements of sleep restriction.

SLEEP HYGIENE

Sleep hygiene should be emphasized in the treatment of any chronic insomnia, including psychophysiological insomnia. Good sleep hygiene includes the following:

1. **Regular sleep time**. Establishing a regular sleep-wake schedule is very important, especially a regular time of arising in the morning, with no more than ± 1 hour deviation from day to day, including weekends. Getting up at 6:00 A.M. on weekdays to go to work and then sleeping in until noon on weekends should be discouraged. Time of arising is an important synchronizer of circadian rhythms, so it should be early enough that the patient does not spend excessive amounts of time in bed in the morning after awakening.
2. **Proper sleep environment**. Special attention should be paid to avoid *temperature extremes* in the bedroom; excessively warm temperatures disturb sleep. It is necessary to specifically inquire about *noise*, because patients may habituate to a noisy sleep environment and may not remember the noise, although it continues to disrupt their sleep pattern. Ensuring that the sleep environment is away from busy streets and away from or properly curtained from bright lights may be helpful. Sleep interruptions should be minimized. Patients who have convinced themselves that they can only sleep with the radio or television on should be discouraged from this practice. While

attention to the radio or TV may prevent their minds from wandering, or may keep them from beginning to worry about other matters, and thus assist with sleep latency, the continuing noise will be more of a disruptive factor during the course of the night. Clock radios that automatically turn themselves off may be useful.

3. **Wind-down time**. Time to wind down prior to sleep is important. Advise patients to stop work at least 30 minutes prior to sleep onset time, and change their activities to something different and nonstressful, such as reading, watching television, or listening to music.

4. **Stimulus control**. This procedure, an important component of sleep hygiene, involves removing from the bedroom all stimuli that are not associated with sleep. The bedroom should be used for sleep, and of course sexual activity (which is often conducive to sleep). Activities such as eating, drinking, arguing, discussing the day's problems, and paying bills should be done elsewhere, because their associated arousal may interfere with sleep onset.

5. **Avoidance of time in bed worrying**. Patients should be encouraged not to remain in bed worrying and fretting about not being able to sleep or worrying about activities that may be planned for the next day. If they find themselves unable to sleep after 30 minutes, they should get up, read, or perform and complete a task, and then return to bed after they note the onset of sleepiness. Remaining in bed trying to fight wakefulness can further aggravate a conditioned arousal to the sleep setting.

6. **Avoidance of alcohol and caffeine**. Caffeine is quite disruptive of nocturnal sleep in many patients, and it has a substantial half-life. Thus it is recommended that caffeine consumption be limited to the forenoon and not be continued after noon. A glass of wine or beer in the evening may help some individuals relax, but regularly having several drinks before bedtime for the express purpose of using the alcohol as a sedative should be discouraged. Alcohol in large doses can substantially disrupt and fragment sleep, and act as a potent REM suppressor, with suppression of REM early in the night, and REM rebound, perhaps accompanied by vivid dreams, in the early

morning hours. *Cigarette smoking* may produce or aggravate insomnia in some patients.

7. **Late tryptophan snack**. A bedtime snack such as a glass of milk, a cookie, a banana, or a similar high-tryptophan food may help promote sleep onset in some patients. L-Tryptophan in doses of 2–4 grams is also occasionally effective, possibly because as a serotonin precursor it acts to stimulate the serotonergic systems thought to underlie sleep-inducing and sleep-maintaining systems. Further information on tryptophan can be found in Chapter 7.

8. **Regular exercise**. Periods of exercise 20–30 minutes long at least 3–4 days a week should be encouraged. Exercise has been shown experimentally to promote slow wave sleep. Exercise should not occur within 3 hours of bedtime, however, because the autonomic arousal accompanying the exercise may serve to delay sleep onset.

SELF-CONTROL TECHNIQUES

Self-control techniques are important because many patients with chronic insomnia experience considerable frustration with the idea that they are not able to control their sleep-wake patterns, and feel out of control when they are unable to sleep at night. Such patients are more comfortable when they are in control of their lives in general, with respect to both daytime activity and sleep. This information can usually be elicited in an interview by direct questioning, and for these patients treatment strategies designed to enhance a sense of self-control should be considered as part of their comprehensive insomnia treatment program. These treatment strategies may include *supportive therapy* aimed at dealing with control issues, the use of *autogenic training*, *relaxation tapes* or training in *progressive relaxation*, or a recommendation that the patient participate in a *meditation* training program that fosters a sense of self-control.

BIOFEEDBACK

Biofeedback treatment that directly teaches patients how to control autonomic functioning may be a useful therapeutic strategy as well (29). Biofeedback may serve the dual function of enhancing a sense of self-control and reducing autonomic arousal. While

EMG and skin temperature biofeedback systems are perhaps the most commonly available forms, EEG theta biofeedback has been shown to be useful in tense, anxious patients with psychophysiological insomnia, and EEG sensorimotor rhythm (SMR) biofeedback has been shown to be useful in patients with psychophysiological insomnia who are not particularly tense or anxious, but who nonetheless have trouble sleeping. SMR biofeedback is at present rarely available, however. Some therapists believe that the patients most likely to benefit from biofeedback will be those individuals who have previously demonstrated the ability to stick to and master difficult challenges (e.g., having achieved success in music as a child or in academic ventures).

SLEEP RESTRICTION

Patients with chronic insomnia frequently wind up spending greater and greater amounts of time in bed getting less and less sleep, such that they may be in bed 10 or more hours and sleeping only 6 hours. Sleep tends to spread out among the hours spent in bed, and this further fragments nocturnal sleep. The principle of sleep restriction is to decrease substantially the time spent in bed, such that sleep will consolidate to that time (30). Restricting time available for sleep results in improved consolidation, which has important benefits in terms of improving actual and perceived sleep quality, as well as improving the patient's subjective sense of self-control over sleep habits, an important consideration. Many chronic insomnia patients will respond quite dramatically to a sleep restriction program, and we believe this type of program should be considered as part of most insomnia treatment regimens. The steps involved include the following:

1. Have the patient maintain a *sleep diary* for at least five nights. This diary should include (a) time to bed at night, (b) estimated time of sleep onset, (c) number and estimated time of awakenings during night, (d) time of final awakening in the morning, and (e) time out of bed. From this five-night sleep diary data, calculate the mean value for estimated total sleep time (TST), and the percent sleep efficiency ([TST/total time in bed] x 100).

2. Set the beginning total time in bed to equal the mean TST. Thus, for example, if the patient's estimate of his or her total sleep time per night averaged over five nights comes to 5½ hours, set the time in bed to no more than 5½ hours, perhaps having the patient go to bed at 12:30 A.M. and get up again at 6:00 A.M. This restriction will result in increased daytime sleepiness the first several days, so the patient may need encouragement to continue with the program.
3. Instruct the patient to call in, usually to an answering machine, every morning while on the program and report his or her sleep data for the previous night, including time to bed, time of awakenings during sleep, time of final awakening, and time out of bed.
4. Calculate TST and sleep efficiency for each night. When mean sleep efficiency for five nights in a row reaches 85% or better, increase time in bed by 15 minutes, by allowing the patient to go to bed 15 minutes earlier. If mean sleep efficiency falls below 85%, decrease time in bed by 15 minutes (but not within the first 10 days of treatment). Naps outside the prescribed time in bed are not allowed.
5. The above procedure is repeated until the patient is maintaining a sleep efficiency of 85% or better and obtaining what he or she considers to be a subjectively adequate amount of nocturnal sleep.

Sleep restriction results in some unavoidable sleepiness at the beginning of the regimen, and not all patients can carry it through. However, those who can have a substantial chance of improving their sleep efficiency. Normally those patients who are going to respond will begin to improve the latter part of the first week, after a few initial days of considerable daytime fatigue as they adjust to the new schedule.

PHARMACOLOGICAL COMPONENTS

Pharmacological components of the insomnia treatment package might include a short-half-life benzodiazepine hypnotic such as triazolam (Halcion) 0.125 mg hs or temazepam (Restoril) 15 mg hs. In the absence of other medical or psychiatric indications, the hypnotic should not be used every night, but rather two to three times per week as occasion arises. Tryptophan is occasionally helpful. The use of hypnotics is considered further in Chapter 7.

In addition to the conventional hypnotic agents, tricyclics often play an important role in the treatment of chronic psychophysiological insomnia (31). Tricyclics are frequently indicated in sleep problems related to affective disorders but are often useful in other insomnias as well. In the experience of a number of clinicians (which has *not* yet included blind controlled studies), a tricyclic can often be of benefit to the patient with chronic sleep maintenance insomnia, or early morning awakening, especially if a degree of dysphoria or depressive affect seems to be present (which appears frequently to be the case in many patients with chronic insomnia). Sedative tricyclics such as amitriptyline, nortriptyline, trimipramine, and doxepin, which are strongly antihistaminic, are often used. Special caution should be taken with patients who have increased risk factors such as cardiac conduction defects, glaucoma, or seizure disorders. A benzodiazepine might be a better first choice in such cases.

In those cases in which tricyclics are indicated, we frequently begin with nortriptyline 25 mg hs, increasing dosage to 75 or more mg hs, with beneficial effects frequently seen within a day or two. If the patient can tolerate the more sedative amitriptyline, beneficial sleep effects may be seen with the first dose.

Several advantages of tricyclics include their low abuse potential and their relative suitability for long-term use. They have associated risks as well, including cardiac conduction problems and greater potential lethality with overdose. They also have the potential to exacerbate nocturnal myoclonus, again emphasizing the importance of accurate initial assessment.

■ RARE CAUSES OF INSOMNIA

This chapter has thus far outlined the large majority of the causes of transient and chronic insomnias. Occasionally, a patient may present with insomnia from one of the following generally rare conditions. There are likely other causes of idiopathic or "primary" insomnia yet to be described.

CHILDHOOD ONSET INSOMNIA

Childhood onset insomnia characterizes a group of patients who have complained of insomnia since early childhood—usually beginning as far back as the patient can remember, with sleep onset and sleep maintenance insomnia (32). Adult patients often remember lying in bed at night for hours being unable to get to or remain asleep, and sometimes getting up in the middle of the night to play, read, etc. Adult symptoms may include significant daytime sleepiness. The etiology of childhood onset insomnia is not clear, although neurophysiological mechanisms are thought to be important; nor is it yet clear that this insomnia is a single entity. Many children with brain or developmental abnormalities experience irregular and interrupted sleep, with a lower sensory threshold. Some childhood onset insomnia patients may represent such children grown up. Polysomnography shows prolonged sleep latency, low sleep efficiency, and low total sleep time; it may also show long REM periods, with lower than normal phasic activity.

The treatment of this disorder should probably include improved sleep hygiene techniques as well as medication, although there is no agreement on which medication is most appropriate. Regestein and Reich (33) describe two childhood onset insomnia patients, both with evidence of some CNS dysfunction, one of whom (with a relatively high percent of Stage 3 and Stage 4 sleep on the PSG) responded favorably to opiates, the other (with a low percent of Stage 3 and Stage 4 sleep on the PSG and other evidence of lack of serotonin production) responded to the serotonergic drug trazodone 200 mg daily. It would seem that no generalization can be offered for this condition; specific etiological factors must be evaluated for each case, with treatment tailored to specific findings.

REM INTERRUPTION INSOMNIA

REM interruption insomnia is characterized by awakenings from REM periods, often relatively early in the period (34). These awakenings result in both insomnia complaints and some apparent REM deprivation. Some patients have complained of nightmares prior to the development of REM awakenings; thus the awakenings might be seen as an effort to ward off the nightmares. Clues to a possible REM interruption insomnia are provided by periodic awakenings with memory of dream content prior to awakenings. The disorder has been conceptualized as primarily psychological in origin, and treatment should be so directed, although an REM-suppressant tricyclic might be appropriate for some patients.

■ REFERENCES

1. Kales A, Soldatos CR, Bixler EO, et al: Rebound insomnia and rebound anxiety: a review. Pharmacology 26:121–137, 1983
2. Busto U, Sellers EM, Naranjo CA, et al: Withdrawal reaction after long term therapeutic use of benzodiazepines. N Engl J Med 315:854–859, 1986
3. Conell LJ, Berlin RM: Withdrawal after substitution of a short-acting for a long-acting benzodiazepine. JAMA 250:2838–2840, 1983
4. Weitzman ED, Czeisler C, Coleman RM, et al: Delayed sleep phase syndrome: a chronobiological disorder error with sleep onset insomnia. Arch Gen Psychiatry 38:737–746, 1981
5. Czeisler CA, Allan JS, Strogatz SH, et al: Bright light resets the human circadian pacemaker independent of the timing of the sleep-wake cycle. Science 233:667–671, 1986
6. Moore-Ede MC, Richardson GS: Medical implications of shift work. Ann Rev Med 36:607–617, 1985
7. Gordon NP, Cleary PD, Parker CE, et al: The prevalence and health impact of shiftwork. Am J Public Health 76:1225–1228, 1986
8. Czeisler CA, Moore-Ede MC, Coleman RM: Rotating shift work schedules that disrupt sleep are improved by applying circadian principles. Science 217:460–463, 1982
9. Ekbom KA: Restless leg syndrome. Neurology (Minn) 10:868–874, 1960
10. Coleman RM, Roffwarg HP, Kennedy SJ, et al: Sleep-wake disorders based on a polysomnographic diagnosis. A national cooperative study. JAMA 247:997–1003, 1982
11. Ancoli-Israel S, Kripke DF, Mason W, et al: Sleep apnea and periodic movements in an aging sample. J Gerontol 40:419–425, 1985
12. Reite M, Higgs L, Reed N: Polysomnographic findings in chronic psychophysiological insomnia. Sleep Research 18:293, 1989

13. Reynolds G, Blake DR, Pall HS, et al: Restless leg syndrome and rheumatoid arthritis. Br Med J 292:639–660, 1986
14. Jacobson JH, Rosenberg RS, Huttenlocher PR, et al: Familial nocturnal cramping. Sleep 9:54–60, 1986
15. Lugaresi E, Cirignotta F, Coccagna G, et al: Nocturnal myoclonus and restless leg syndrome, in Advances in Neurology, Vol 43, Myoclonus. Edited by Fahn S, et al. New York, Raven Press, 1986, pp 295–307
16. Wechsler LR, Stakes JW, Shahani BT, et al: Periodic leg movements of sleep (nocturnal myoclonus): an electrophysiological study. Ann Neurol 19:168–173, 1986
17. Spillane JD, Nethan PW, Kelly RE, et al: Painful legs and moving toes. Brain 94:541–556, 1971
18. Myers BA, Klerman GL, Hartmann E: Nocturnal cataclysms with myoclonus: a new side effect of clomipramine. Am J Psychiatry 143:1490–1491, 1986
19. Broughton R, Tolentino MA, Krelina M: Excessive fragmentary myoclonus in NREM sleep: a report of 38 cases. Electroencephalogr Clin Neurophysiol 61:123–133, 1985
20. Mitler MM, Browman CP, Menn SJ, et al: Nocturnal myoclonus: treatment efficacy of clonazepam and temazepam. Sleep 9:385–392, 1986
21. Guilleminault C, Flagg W: Effects of baclofen on sleep-related periodic leg movements. Ann Neurol 15:234–239, 1984
22. Hening WA, Walters A, Kavey N, et al: Dyskinesias while awake and periodic movements in sleep in restless legs syndrome: treatment with opioids. Neurology 36:1363–1366, 1986
23. Ancoli-Israel S, Seifert AR, Lemon M: Thermal biofeedback and periodic movements in sleep: patients' subjective reports and a case study. Biofeedback Self Regul 11:177–188, 1986
24. Ancoli-Israel S, Kripke DF, Mason W: Characteristics of obstructive and central sleep apnea in the elderly: an interim report. Biol Psychiatry 22:741–750, 1987
25. White DP: Central sleep apnea. Med Clin North Am 69:1205–1219, 1985
26. Lugaresi E, Zucconi M, Bixler EO: Epidemiology of sleep disorders. Psychiatr Ann 17:446–453, 1987
27. Sewitch DE: Slow wave sleep deficiency insomnia: a problem in thermo-downregulation at sleep onset. Psychophysiology 24:200–215, 1987
28. Healey ES, Kales A, Monroe L, et al: Onset of insomnia: role of life stress events. Psychosom Med 43:439–451, 1981

29. Hauri PJ, Percy L, Hellekson C, et al: The treatment of psychophysiological insomnia with biofeedback: a replication study. Biofeedback Self Regul 7:223–235, 1983
30. Spielman AJ, Saskin P, Thorpy MJ: Treatment of chronic insomnia by restriction of time in bed. Sleep 10:45–56, 1987
31. Ware JC: Tricyclic antidepressants in the treatment of insomnia. J Clin Psychiatry 44:25–28, 1983
32. Hauri P, Olmstead E: Childhood-onset insomnia. Sleep 3:59–65, 1980
33. Regestein QR, Reich P: Incapacitating childhood-onset insomnia. Compr Psychiatry 24:244–248, 1983
34. Greenberg R: Dream interruption insomnia. J Nerv Ment Dis 144:18–21, 1967

■ ADDITIONAL READINGS

Kales A, Kales JD: Evaluation and Treatment of Insomnia. New York, Oxford University Press, 1984

Williams RL, Karacan I, Moore CA (eds): Sleep Disorders: Diagnosis and Treatment, 2nd Edition. New York, John Wiley, 1988

4 EXCESSIVE SLEEPINESS DISORDERS

■ EVALUATION OF EXCESSIVE DAYTIME SLEEPINESS

Excessive daytime sleepiness (EDS) is a relatively common complaint, found in 1% of inpatients and over 4% of industrial workers. EDS has a wide spectrum of presentation, ranging from mild sleepiness through decrements in daytime performance due to extreme sleepiness, perhaps with "microsleeps," to industrial or motor vehicle accidents due to uncontrollable sleep attacks. True EDS symptoms must be differentiated from fatigue, tiredness, and lack of motivation that are also quite common and often associated with depression and various insomnias.

EDS is rarely found in preadolescent children, but when present it must be taken seriously as a possible indicator of a sleep apnea disorder. Significant increases in EDS may accompany adolescence, at which point it may be secondary to insufficient nocturnal sleep, or may herald the emergence of more serious problems such as narcolepsy or depression. College students and young adults often complain of EDS, but poor sleep habits and insufficient nocturnal sleep are often the culprits. In adults, EDS symptoms may result from a variety of causes ranging from medical disorders to poor sleep habits. EDS symptoms must be taken seriously and evaluated both quickly and comprehensively because they may represent potentially serious medical disorders in need of treatment, and because the symptoms themselves can have serious consequences, such as motor vehicle accidents. Frequent causes of EDS are listed in Table 4-1.

The evaluation of EDS begins with a good history of daytime function. The patient should be questioned about alertness throughout the day, emphasizing times when sleep may be most likely, such as in boring sedentary situations. The use of naps (frequency, duration, and effect on alertness) should be explored. Specific questions concerning uncontrollable sleepiness when doing activities such as eating, walking, talking, driving, or operat-

TABLE 4-1. **Frequent causes of excessive daytime sleepiness**

Sleep apnea and other sleep-related breathing disorders
Narcolepsy
Idiopathic CNS hypersomnolence
Psychiatric disorders
Periodic limb movements of sleep
Chronic use of drugs or alcohol
Other medical disorders
Periodic hypersomnias (Kleine-Levin syndrome and menstruation-associated hypersomnia)
Insufficient sleep
Sleep-wake cycle disorder
Long sleeper

ing equipment should be asked. Subtle diminution in alertness manifested by decrements in performance at work, difficulty with memory, or confusional spells should be queried. The use of caffeine and other stimulants (including over-the-counter products) may indicate the presence of an underlying EDS disorder. All medications used should be reviewed with regard to their possible sedating or alerting side effects. In addition, the onset, duration, and possible periodicity of daytime sleepiness are of diagnostic value. A family history with regard to symptoms of excessive somnolence and cataplexy should be obtained.

In children, complaints of EDS may first emerge from the classroom, as the child falls asleep in school or fails to pay attention. Such children are often first thought to be lazy. Again, a complete description of the symptoms, perhaps obtained from the teacher, is important, as well as appropriate medical and family history.

The degree of daytime alertness may be subjectively quantified with rating scales such as the Stanford Sleepiness Scale (1), or objectively quantified with the multiple sleep latency test (MSLT), as described in Chapter 1.

A decision tree for the evaluation of an EDS complaint is illustrated in Figure 4-1. This tree suggests that insufficient sleep resulting from either an insomnia disorder or poor sleep hygiene or habits should be considered first. If these causes seem unlikely, then one should explore EDS secondary to a sleep-related breathing disorder, narcolepsy, or psychiatric disorder, as well as rare causes of EDS. The decision tree illustrated in Figure 4-1 is provided only as a guide for the evaluation of an EDS complaint. The evaluation process should not stop with the first evidence suggesting an etiology, because not infrequently more than one cause may be operative, such as is the case with obstructive sleep apnea in a patient with previously undiagnosed narcolepsy. The initial evaluation should consider all possibilities the first time around.

Most patients with an EDS complaint will require a polysomnogram (PSG) and MSLT as a part of the diagnostic evaluation. Exceptions would be those patients whose complaints seem clearly related to insufficient nocturnal sleep or poor sleep habits, or to a psychiatric disorder that can be separately treated.

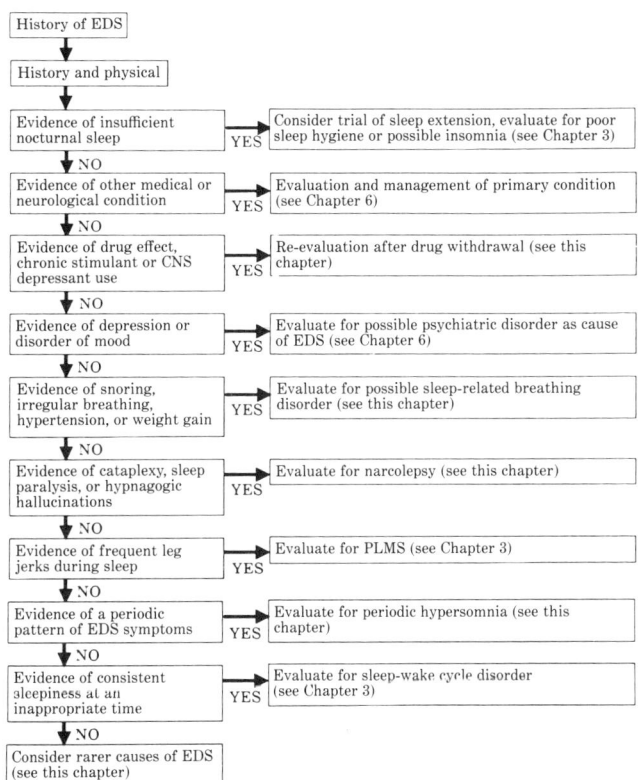

FIGURE 4-1. **Decision tree for evaluation of excessive daytime sleepiness (EDS) complaint.**

In these cases, the effects of treatment of the underlying disorder on the EDS complaint should be monitored. If the EDS symptoms improve with the underlying disorder, further sleep workup may not be needed. If these symptoms do not improve, a PSG and MSLT may still be required.

■ NARCOLEPSY

PRESENTING COMPLAINTS

- Excessive daytime sleepiness
- Episodes of irresistible sleepiness
- Paroxysmal muscle weakness, often elicited by emotion or surprise (cataplexy)
- Temporary inability to initiate motor movement preceding sleep or upon awakening (sleep paralysis)
- Hypnagogic hallucinations
- Automatic behavior
- Disturbed nocturnal sleep

CLINICAL PRESENTATION

Excessive daytime sleepiness, the hallmark of narcolepsy, typically begins between ages 10 and 30. EDS may begin being manifested as a greater tendency to fall asleep in situations where many people may fall asleep, such as in classes or lectures, after eating, while riding in cars, in warm environments, or in situations where a person is excessively tired. The pathological aspect of narcolepsy may become more apparent after detecting frequent dozing off, as well as falling asleep, in unusual circumstances such as standing up, walking, during physical exercise, or during painful or typically stimulating activities.

Typical warning signals of the onset of a "sleep attack" may be tiredness, heaviness of limbs, inability to focus the eyes, inability to keep eyes open, loss of neck muscle tone or "head bobbing," and occasionally hypnagogic hallucinations. Most sleep episodes come on gradually and there is enough warning for the narcoleptic person to get in a safe position or pull a car over to the side of the road before having an accident. Eventually, however, the narcoleptic individual may succumb to sleep, which lasts 10 to 30 minutes and will most frequently be followed by a short period of improved alertness and a feeling of being refreshed. The most dangerous symptom of narcolepsy is the sudden onset of sleep with no prior warning, which can result in accidents while driving or at work. Such sudden onset accompanies relatively few episodes of sleepiness; nonetheless, it has been reported that 48% of narcoleptic individuals have fallen asleep while driving (2).

Frequency of daytime naps is widely variable among narcoleptic individuals, but it is generally reported to be in the range of one to eight per day. In addition to these irresistible periods of sleep, narcoleptic individuals will frequently have very brief microsleeps throughout the day, as well as periods of subwakefulness or significantly impaired alertness.

There is evidence that some narcoleptic individuals have a rhythmicity to their tendency toward sleepiness during the daytime that may be similar to the approximately 90-minute periodicity of REM sleep during nocturnal sleep. For many of these individuals it is easier to fight off early morning attacks of sleepiness, but as the day goes on, they may be less and less able to avoid napping.

Although remissions have been reported, the overall course of the illness tends to show clinical stability or mild deterioration. There is no cure for narcolepsy, but in most cases the symptoms can be adequately managed.

The classic *narcoleptic tetrad* includes EDS, as well as the symptoms cataplexy, sleep paralysis, and hypnagogic hallucinations. It is estimated that only 10–15% of narcoleptic individuals display the full tetrad of symptoms, and members of the same family can exhibit different traits within the tetrad.

Cataplexy is the sudden partial or complete loss of muscle tone in response to sudden emotional stimuli such as laughter, anger, surprise, or joy. Frequently, loss of tone will be confined to face, neck, and limb muscles, but occasionally a generalized cataplexy with complete skeletal muscle atonia and paralysis can occur. During the episode the subject will have loss of tendon reflexes and occasionally a positive Babinski sign and loss of pupillary light reaction. These episodes usually last no more than a few seconds and usually do not result in injury to the patient or loss of consciousness. If prolonged (i.e., lasting up to a minute), full-blown REM sleep will ensue.

Cataplectic attacks can vary in frequency from once in many years to 15–20 times per day. Approximately 70% of all narcoleptic individuals will suffer from occasional cataplexy; 10–20% of subjects will have improvement over time, and many can learn to diminish the frequency of episodes by avoiding sudden excitement or by tensing muscles during situations that might trigger the cataplexy. Cataplexy most often appears several years after the onset of EDS, with individual case onsets reported as much as 30 years later.

Sleep paralysis occurs in about 25% of narcoleptic individuals. A typical patient will complain that once or twice per week, usually at the time of sleep onset, there will be a period when mental alertness is maintained but the subject is paralyzed except for respiratory and eye musculature. The episodes seem to be terminated by noises, external stimuli, or the patient falling asleep. Occasionally, episodes will also occur upon morning awakening.

Hypnagogic hallucinations consist of vivid auditory, somasthetic, or visual dream-like hallucinations usually occurring at sleep onset. These episodes, which typically last only a few minutes, are a frequent accompaniment of sleep paralysis and are present in about 30% of narcoleptic individuals. Hypnagogic hallucinations and sleep paralysis are not unique to narcolepsy, however, as described in Chapter 5.

Automatic behavior is present in 20–40% of narcoleptic individuals. These episodes often consist of memory lapses, repetitive meaningless behaviors, and spoken phrases or written sentences totally out of previous context. Automatic behavior frequently shows up while driving, with long periods of time apparently forgotten, or by traveling to the wrong destination for no apparent reason. Such episodes can also contribute to illegal driving behavior, car accidents, and poor work performance.

Sleep drunkenness consists of mental clouding and confusion for the first 30–60 minutes after morning awakening. This symptom is a characteristic of approximately 10% of narcoleptic individuals.

The nocturnal sleep of most narcoleptic individuals is often significantly disrupted. These individuals are prone to frequent nocturnal spontaneous arousals as well as a greater incidence of periodic limb movements of sleep (PLMS) and sleep apnea (3).

INCIDENCE

The prevalence of narcolepsy has been estimated to be between 0.05 and 0.07% of the population (4). One third of all narcoleptic individuals will have a positive family history, and relatives of narcoleptic persons have a 60-fold greater chance of developing narcolepsy themselves.

ETIOLOGY AND PATHOPHYSIOLOGY

Many of the daytime symptoms of narcolepsy seem to be secondary to a pathological intrusion of REM sleep physiology into wakefulness. REM sleep physiology includes a descending inhibition of neuronal input to striated muscle, which results in the loss of muscle tone seen in cataplexy and the paralysis seen in sleep paralysis. Hypnagogic hallucinations appear related to dream-like mentation accompanying REM sleep. Whether there may also be an associated disturbance of function of non-REM sleep systems is not clear. Associated abnormalities in catecholamine systems thought to be involved in the control of REM and non-REM sleep have been sought, both in humans and in canine models of narcolepsy, but clear findings are elusive.

Studies in a canine model of narcolepsy have suggested that central α-1-adrenergic receptors may play an important role in controlling both narcolepsy and cataplexy. Prazosin, a selective α-1-adrenergic receptor blocker, substantially aggravates cataplexy in narcoleptic dogs, whereas treatment with the α-1 agonist methoxamine ameliorates it (5).

Almost all narcoleptic individuals have in common the major histocompatibility antigen HLA-DR2. The familial incidence of narcolepsy, in addition to the strong relationship of narcolepsy with HLA-DR2, suggests that a genetic defect occurs in narcoleptic individuals that manifests itself in either a neurochemical or an immunological pathway. Some narcoleptic subjects show oligoclonal bands or raised immunoglobulin concentrations in the cerebrospinal fluid, suggesting that narcolepsy may be an immune-mediated disorder for which the HLA-DR2 antigen represents a genetic susceptibility (6). Narcoleptic patients with

HLA-DR2 can be differentiated from healthy individuals with HLA-DR2 by detecting the presence of HLA-DQ$_b$ chain DNA restriction fragments (7).

Complicating the picture is that all narcolepsy cases do not fit into the idiopathic variety but at times seem to be secondary to infections, tumors, head trauma, and possibly endocrine disorders. Some of these cases may not have been true narcolepsy, however, but rather other hypersomnia disorders, or they may have been related to narcolepsy only by coincidence. Postinfectious narcolepsy could be a situation in which the immune system's response to a specific antigen may be a causative factor for the onset of narcolepsy. The final answers to such possible relationships await further research.

LABORATORY FINDINGS

Narcolepsy is one of the few sleep disorders for which sleep laboratory findings are specific, demonstrating both excessive sleepiness and a greater than normal tendency for REM sleep. The MSLT will most often demonstrate an abnormally short mean sleep latency (5 minutes or less) for five nap periods, and this, in addition to the presence of two or more sleep onset REM periods (REM sleep within 10 minutes of sleep onset) on the MSLT, is considered diagnostic of narcolepsy. Typical MSLT findings from a group of narcoleptic patients are shown in Figure 4-2. A nocturnal PSG should precede the MSLT to ensure that the preceding night's sleep had not been severely abnormal (e.g., severe sleep apnea). It is common to find moderate sleep disturbances on the preceding night's PSG, however, in the form of myoclonus, mild sleep apnea, and frequent awakenings. Abnormally short REM latencies will not necessarily be seen on the PSG.

DIFFERENTIAL DIAGNOSIS

Narcolepsy is strongly suggested by the presence of the narcoleptic tetrad, especially EDS and cataplexy, and further supported by a positive family history. The diagnosis can be confirmed by an MSLT with average sleep latency under 5 minutes and two sleep onset REM periods, and further supported by presence of HLA-

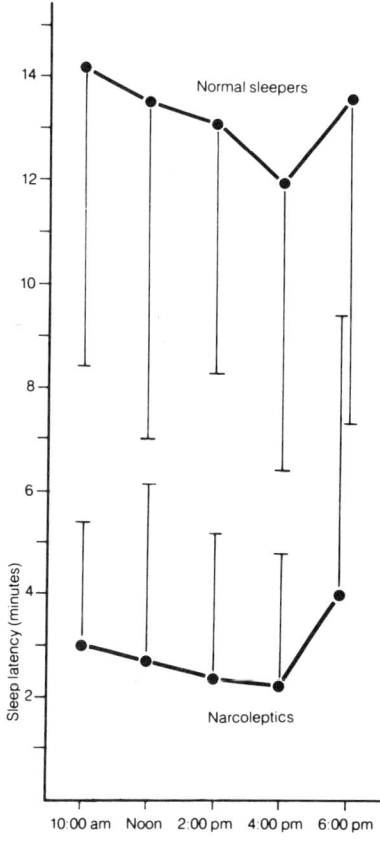

●―● = means
T = standard deviation

FIGURE 4-2. **Typical MSLT findings for group of narcoleptic patients.**
These patients have shorter sleep latencies than do non-narcoleptic sleepers on each of the five naps comprising the MSLT. Reprinted, with permission, from Hauri P: The Sleep Disorders. Kalamazoo, MI, The Upjohn Company, 1982. Copyright 1982, Scope Publications, The Upjohn Company.

DR2 antigen. The presence of a borderline MSLT should not absolutely eliminate the diagnosis of narcolepsy if this disorder is still strongly suspected clinically. The onset of the symptoms of narcolepsy can be variable, and it is likely that there is somewhat of a normal distribution of sleep latencies and presence of sleep onset REM periods within narcoleptic individuals. Narcoleptic patients who have negative MSLT results, if studied more than once, will frequently show positive findings on subsequent studies.

The clinician must remember that it is not uncommon for individuals to feign narcolepsy to obtain stimulants. For this reason, it may be important to do urine drug screens on suspected individuals to ensure that sleep latency is not shortened by the abuse of sedatives or withdrawal from stimulants. Similarly, even though the presence of cataplexy is pathognomonic for the diagnosis of narcolepsy, this is a self-reported symptom. Thus, the diagnosis should be confirmed by sleep laboratory studies for protection of both patient and physician.

Other causes of EDS, listed in Table 4-1, should be excluded before a final diagnosis of narcolepsy is made. It is, of course, possible for more than one cause of EDS to coexist, which would have treatment implications.

TREATMENT

Comprehensive therapy for the narcoleptic patient includes both behavioral and pharmacological facets. It is very important to keep in mind the chronicity of the disorder, as well as its pervasive effects on occupational, emotional, social, and physical functioning. Of prime importance should be helping to prevent the patient from falling asleep while driving or in a dangerous work setting.

BEHAVIORAL TREATMENT COMPONENTS

1. *Optimal sleep hygiene* to maximize quality and quantity of nocturnal sleep (see Chapter 3 for details). It is especially important for the narcoleptic patient to strive for getting a restful night's sleep by keeping regular bedtime and arising time; having a bedroom that is cool, comfortable, and free of

excessive noise, light, or distraction; and keeping stimulant dosages early enough in the day to avoid interference with sleep onset, or excessive arousals. Avoidance of alcohol should be promoted and sedatives or tranquilizers should be used only as specifically warranted for treatment of concomitant sleep problems such as periodic leg movements or poorly consolidated nocturnal sleep. Exercise can both increase the depth of nocturnal sleep and provide a temporary way to shake off drowsiness.
2. *Brief regularly scheduled daytime naps* in the range of 15–30 minutes. These naps have been shown to be an effective adjunctive treatment for sleepiness in narcoleptic patients.
3. *Education* of the patient, family, teachers, and employer regarding the treatment and the natural history of this illness. A chronic illness can be very discouraging and disruptive for both patient and family. It is especially important that an employer or teacher is aware of the nature of the illness and especially the need to make use of daytime naps. The physician may need to collaborate with the employer to explain both the napping and the need for stimulant medication.

PHARMACOLOGICAL TREATMENT COMPONENTS

The following pharmacological components are designed to target (a) daytime sleepiness, (b) cataplexy, and (c) associated symptoms. Daytime sleepiness is generally managed by CNS stimulants, with *pemoline*, *methylphenidate*, and *dextroamphetamine* most commonly used in the United States.

Pemoline is a relatively mild stimulant that can be started at a dosage of 37.5 mg once a day in the morning or 18.75 mg in the morning and again at noon. The advantages of pemoline include few side effects, low addiction potential, and the possibility of once-daily morning dosage. Because of its very long half-life it may need to accumulate in the system for a few days to reach its full effectiveness. Dosages can be increased to as high as 300 mg per day if necessary, or until untoward side effects develop.

Methylphenidate, in a dose range of 10–60 mg per day, is the drug of choice for those patients not responding to pemoline, and provides very good relief in better than 75% of patients using it. In general, it tends to have a stimulant potency nearly equal to that of dextroamphetamine, but with less of a tendency to cause anorexia and increases in heart rate and blood pressure. The drug is commonly given in two to three divided doses per day. The onset of action is within 30–60 minutes, reaching peak effectiveness in 2–4 hours after administration. Dosage times are usually tailored to the patient's typical daily regimen, with the patient often taking dosages after brief naps, to allow maximal wakefulness during work periods or to provide maximal alertness during critical situations such as driving or attending important social events. After defining a sufficient dose the majority of patients can stabilize at one dosage level for many years. Visual hallucinosis or psychosis is a rare side effect of both methylphenidate and dextroamphetamine and amphetamine.

Dextroamphetamine can be prescribed at similar dosages and timing as those used with methylphenidate. Most patients will experience dextroamphetamine as slightly more potent than methylphenidate and will prefer its usage. There is a great deal of cross-tolerance between the two drugs, but select patients will prefer a monthly alternation between methylphenidate and dextroamphetamine, and over a period of years they will report maximal effectiveness for the first 2 weeks after each switch.

Protriptyline is a mildly stimulating tricyclic that can very mildly increase alertness as well as block cataplexy. Some patients find benefit in the use of protriptyline 5–30 mg per day, either alone, in milder cases, or as an adjunct to the CNS stimulants (8).

A number of other compounds have been used experimentally or are available for foreign usage. These compounds include γ-hydroxybutyrate, propranolol, mazindol, codeine, diethylpropion, phentermine, fencamfamine, and select monoamine oxidase inhibitors. Their efficacy and specificity generally have yet to be documented in well-controlled double-blind studies.

Cataplexy and sleep paralysis can be effectively treated with tricyclics, which are potent REM suppressors, in two-thirds of narcoleptic patients. Most commonly used are imipramine 10–100 mg per day, desipramine 10–100 mg per day, or protriptyline 5–30 mg per day. The dosages are smaller than that needed for an antidepressant effect, and because of their long-acting nature, these drugs can usually be given once a day at any time. For those who feel some drowsiness secondary to imipramine, the drug can be used at bedtime. In fact, some patients report that this helps with nocturnal sleep as well as blocks their cataplexy.

Difficult cases of cataplexy have been reported to be successfully treated with clonazepam 1–4 mg per day, fluoxetine 20–60 mg per day, femoxetine 600 mg per day, phenelzine 15–90 mg per day, clonidine 0.2 mg per day, γ-hydroxybutyrate 2–4 g per day given at night in divided doses, and viloxazine 50–200 mg per day.

Ancillary symptoms in many narcoleptic patients include disturbed nocturnal sleep, which is in part characterized by spontaneous arousals, PLMS, and sleep apnea. The use of a short- to intermediate-acting benzodiazepine such as triazolam or temazepam may help consolidate sleep and decrease arousals resulting from myoclonic events. Sedatives should not be used if apnea is present. If a tricyclic is used for cataplexy, one must make sure that this does not aggravate myoclonus during the night. For those with a moderate degree of sleep apnea, use of the tricyclic may help cataplexy and reduce sleep apnea, in addition to offering some nighttime sedation.

Some narcoleptic patients experience a significant degree of depression along with their illness. It is important to give the patient an opportunity to talk about the effects the illness has on his or her life, and this may best be done by arranging for formal psychotherapy. If tricyclic antidepressants are necessary in full dosages, one must make sure that the sedative effects do not interfere with control of the daytime sleepiness of the narcolepsy.

■ HYPERSOMNIA DUE TO SLEEP-RELATED BREATHING DISORDERS

In this section we consider primarily the sleep-related breathing disorders that result in symptoms of EDS, i.e., the obstructive apneas, as well as chronic obstructive pulmonary disease (COPD), whose symptoms can be significantly exacerbated during sleep. Central sleep apnea, which usually presents as insomnia, is covered in Chapter 3.

PRESENTING COMPLAINTS

- Excessive daytime sleepiness
- Heavy snoring, sometimes followed by a resuscitative snort
- Restless sleep
- Morning headaches
- Depression, intellectual deterioration, and personality change
- Impotence
- Enuresis
- Decline in school performance in children

CLINICAL PRESENTATION

Patients with sleep apnea usually complain of EDS. Daytime sleepiness varies greatly in different individuals, and frequently is minimized. Excessive sleepiness can be totally denied or may be so severe that it impairs the patient's ability to work or drive. The naps that apneic patients take generally are not very refreshing.

Persons with sleep apnea generally snore, often so loudly that it is disruptive to others sleeping in the same household. Bed partners often note that the patient has repetitive episodes of gradually increasing snoring, followed by a silent pause, which in turn is followed by a loud gasp or inspiratory snort. Violent body movements sometimes accompany this resumption of air flow. The patient with obstructive apnea usually is unaware of any difficulty breathing, or of the excessive body movements. Additional complaints include morning headaches, restless sleep, and arising with a sore throat.

Psychiatric symptoms, including depression, or evidence of memory impairment may be the presenting symptoms of sleep apnea. Impotence, nocturnal seizures, and enuresis are less commonly seen. More disturbing presentations of sleep apnea syndromes include automobile or machine accidents due to falling asleep. In children, a decline in school performance (which may be inappropriately attributed to laziness) may be a presenting symptom.

Approximately 50% of adults with obstructive sleep apnea have coexistent hypertension. Approximately 70% of patients with sleep apnea are at least 20% overweight (9).

A complaint of EDS may also be found in individuals with alveolar hypoventilation, in whom, however, the history of heavy snoring and restless sleep may be absent. Other medical conditions that may impair ventilation, such as poliomyelitis, myotonic dystrophy, obesity, or thoracic wall abnormalities, may be present in such patients.

Patients with primary pulmonary diseases such as COPD or cystic fibrosis can have episodes of hypoxemia, obstructive apneas, or both, when sleeping. Patients with reactive airways disease can complain of increased wheezing, cough, or shortness of breath during the night. They may have disrupted sleep with frequent prolonged arousals, and may complain of daytime fatigue and sleepiness as well.

PATHOPHYSIOLOGY AND ETIOLOGY

APNEA

The process of ventilation is based on air flowing down a gradient of pressure. During inspiration the diaphragm and chest wall muscles generate a large negative intrapleural pressure. This negative pressure causes expansion of the lung parenchyma, and is transmitted as well to the various sized airways. The patency of the oropharyngeal airway depends on pharyngeal dilators to counteract the large negative pressure generated during inspiration. There is a complex neuromuscular mechanism involving the soft palate, the pharyngeal walls, and the tongue, that is activated in a phasic fashion to maintain airway patency. Processes that decrease this neuromuscular activity, such as the muscular hypotonia characteristic of sleep, can allow oropharyngeal airway collapse to occur. The fact that not everyone who sleeps, and thus develops oropharyngeal hypotonia, has upper airway collapse suggests that other coexistent conditions must be present. Current evidence suggests that the majority of patients with sleep apnea have a congenitally small oropharyngeal airway. Other more obvious causes of airway obstruction (e.g., micrognathia, retrognathia, adenotonsillar hypertrophy, nasal obstruction, large uvula, macroglossia, or malignancy) can also contribute to obstructive apnea. It appears that for many patients muscle hypotonia in conjunction with a narrowed airway permits the obstruction to occur.

In children, obstructive apnea is most often secondary to enlargement of tonsils, adenoids, or other lymphoid tissue in the oropharynx, although craniofacial abnormalities such as mandibular hypoplasia can result in obstructive apnea.

The consequences of repetitive episodes of apnea fall into two general categories: medical effects and the effects on sleep itself. Cessation of airflow can lead to oxygen desaturation. The degree of the desaturation depends on the duration of the respiratory event, the O_2 saturation at the beginning of the event, and the lung volume at the time of the event. Oxygen desaturation will be most severe when the apneic event is very long, when the baseline O_2 saturation is already low (i.e., on the steep portion of the oxyhemoglobin dissociation curve), and when the patient has a low lung volume.

Systemic and pulmonary arterial pressures increase during apneic events, and repetitive apneic events can cause a stepwise increase in both these pressures. Once airflow is resumed, these pressures usually return to normal. Recent data indicate that there may be a high incidence of unsuspected sleep apnea in patients with essential hypertension and no specific sleep complaints (10). This finding suggests that sleep apnea may be a contributory factor in chronic hypertension. Cardiac dysrhythmias have been noted to occur with respiratory events. The most common finding is of sinus variability with repetitive episodes of relative bradycardia (during the obstruction), followed by an increased heart rate (during the resumption of airflow)—the so-called "brady-tachycardia." Other dysrhythmias, less commonly seen, include sinus arrest, atrioventricular blocks, ventricular ectopy, and ventricular tachycardia. The frequency of dysrhythmias decreases with adequate treatment of the apnea.

Sleep apnea can also have severely disruptive effects on sleep itself. The termination of a respiratory event often requires a partial arousal from sleep. As a result, sleep for an apneic patient may be quite fragmented, consisting of short periods of light sleep interrupted by frequent arousals. These arousals are often accompanied by an increase in muscular activity manifested by muscle jerks and more complete body movements, described as "restless" sleep.

PRIMARY PULMONARY DISORDERS

Patients with primary pulmonary disorders such as COPD or cystic fibrosis, especially those with CO_2 retention (i.e., the "Blue Bloater"), often experience transient episodes of severe nocturnal hypoxemia. Such patients depend more than typically healthy individuals on the accessory muscles of respiration for their ventilation. During REM sleep the hypotonia of the intercostal and accessory muscles may lead to smaller tidal volumes and decreased minute ventilation. Functional residual capacity is also reduced during REM sleep. Ventilation perfusion mismatching during REM sleep has been hypothesized as well to contribute to O_2 desaturation. Cardiac arrhythmias and elevation in pulmonary artery pressure have been observed during these episodes of hypoxemia. There is a subgroup of patients with chronic pulmonary disease who have coexistent sleep apnea. The combination of these two conditions can lead to profound O_2 desaturation, especially during REM sleep.

Patients with asthma may have an exaggerated nocturnal bronchoconstriction that can lead to increasing symptomatology during the night.

INCIDENCE

Sleep apnea has been estimated to occur in 1–3% of the general population. Additionally, it is estimated that 19% of women and 30% of men are chronic heavy snorers. Sleep apnea can occur in all age groups and both sexes but is most common in middle-aged males.

LABORATORY FINDINGS

An apnea is defined as the cessation of airflow for at least 10 seconds. Three types of apnea have been described: central, obstructive, and mixed. A central apnea (Figure 4-3) occurs when there is lack of respiratory effort by the diaphragm and hence no airflow. An obstructive apnea (Figure 4-4) is present when respiratory effort occurs but no airflow results. A mixed apnea (Figure 4-5) is a combination of both central and obstructive components consisting of an initial central event with cessation of respiratory effort, followed by an interval of effort without airflow, the airway

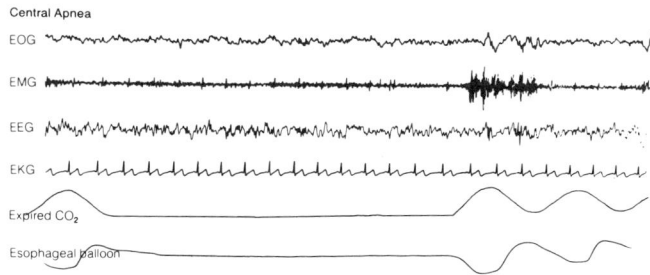

FIGURE 4-3. Central apnea.
Polysomnographic characteristics include absence of both air flow, indicated by no change in expired air CO_2, and respiratory effort, indicated by absence of change in esophageal balloon pressure. Reprinted, with permission, from Hauri P: The Sleep Disorders. Kalamazoo, MI, The Upjohn Company, 1982. Copyright 1982, Scope Publications, The Upjohn Company.

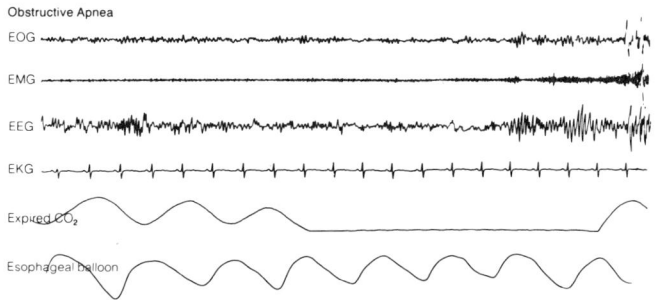

FIGURE 4-4. Obstructive apnea.
Polysomnographic characteristics include absence of air flow, indicated by no change in expired air CO_2, in the presence of continued respiratory effort. Reprinted, with permission, from Hauri P: The Sleep Disorders. Kalamazoo, MI, The Upjohn Company, 1982. Copyright 1982, Scope Publications, The Upjohn Company.

having closed during the central event. In some patients with obstructive apnea, a "paradoxical" motion of the chest wall is seen. In these patients the large negative intrapleural pressure created by the diaphragm causes the chest wall to retract during

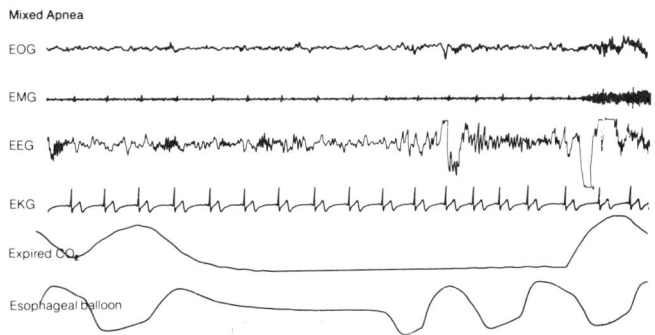

FIGURE 4-5. **Mixed apnea.**
Polysomnographic characteristics include initial absence of both air flow and effort, followed by resumption of effort but, initially, not air flow. Reprinted, with permission, from Hauri P: The Sleep Disorders. Kalamazoo, MI, The Upjohn Company, 1982. Copyright 1982, Scope Publications, The Upjohn Company.

times of airway obstruction. The polysomnographic tracing shows a "phase reverse" of the thoracic motion in relation to abdominal motion at these times.

An apnea index (AI, the number of apneas per 60 minutes of sleep time) of 5 to 8 is probably the upper limit of normality in young adults. Some studies have suggested that older patients may have as many as 17 respiratory events per hour, with only minimal decrements in daytime alertness as measured by the MSLT. Whether sleep apnea of this degree is associated with other physiological consequences is not yet known.

A decrease, but not total cessation, of airflow that lasts at least 10 seconds is termed a "hypopnea." Both apneas and hypopneas can lead to the same end results: oxygen desaturation and arousals. Because of these common effects, both apneas and hypopneas may be added together and described as either the Respiratory Disturbance Index (RDI) or the Apnea-Hypopnea Index (AHI), equaling the sum of the apneas and hypopneas experienced per total number of hours of sleep.

Sleep architecture is often abnormal in patients with apnea, showing fragmented sleep with frequent arousals, and decreased

Stage 3, Stage 4, and REM sleep, as well as cardiac arrhythmias, leg jerks, and body movements and arousals. Sleep often consists predominantly of Stage 1 and Stage 2 sleep. An MSLT the day after the PSG can help quantify the severity of EDS in sleep apnea syndromes.

Patients with sleep-related hypoxemia (e.g., up to 70–80% oxygen saturation) due to nonapneic causes (e.g., COPD patients) will show prolonged episodes of hypoxemia, especially in REM sleep (11). The pattern of desaturation recorded by the oximeter will show a persistently low O_2 saturation rather than a consistently changing saturation typical of repetitive apneic events.

Patients with nocturnal asthma can show a decrement in their flow rates (measured as forced expiratory volume over a 1-second interval [FEV_1], i.e., peak flow rate) if these are measured throughout the night. These patients often complain of nocturnal wheezing and restless sleep (12). Their sleep is inefficient, with frequent and prolonged awakenings.

DIFFERENTIAL DIAGNOSIS

Nocturnal polysomnography is required for proper assessment of sleep-related breathing disorders. Studies of breathing during short daytime naps are not adequate for proper diagnosis because all sleep stages may not be obtained. Breathing disorders are not uniformly present during sleep, tending instead to wax and wane, and frequently becoming more severe during early morning hours. Polysomnographic recording should be sufficient to assess sleep stage, respiratory effort and air flow, tibialis anterior EMG, oximetry, and snoring sounds. It is important to observe if apneas are related to sleep position (e.g., supine vs. sleeping on the side).

EDS due to sleep apnea can usually be differentiated from EDS due to narcolepsy on clinical grounds by the age of onset and the lack of cataplexy, hypnagogic hallucinations, and sleep paralysis, as well as the presence of snoring, morning headaches, and naps that are not refreshing. The presence of hypertension or polycythemia also raises suspicion of a sleep-related breathing disorder.

EDS secondary to depression is more common in adolescents, in whom significant sleep apnea is unusual. Because depression in adults can also be associated with hypersomnolence, and sleep apnea can have depression as a major symptom, the diagnosis is more complicated and requires careful evaluation of both components. Both syndromes may, of course, coexist.

A differentiation of sleep apnea from other chronic causes of excessive somnolence (e.g., idiopathic CNS hypersomnolence, chronic drug dependence, nocturnal myoclonus) often depends on a nocturnal PSG as well as other laboratory tests (e.g., thyroid function, drug screen) and clinical evaluations (e.g., psychiatric interviews). Definite diagnosis of patients with nocturnal hypoxemia due to nonapneic causes begins by ruling out apnea with a PSG, and may then require other pulmonary function tests (e.g., basic spirometry, tests of ventilatory drive, bronchial reactivity).

TREATMENT

APNEA

Treatment ranges from the relatively noninvasive approach, with concurrent slower and less predictable effect, to the invasive approach, with rapid onset and more predictable course. As a rule of thumb, treatment should be tailored to the severity of the disorder, as suggested by the clinical and sleep laboratory evaluation. A schema to help plan treatment is illustrated in Table 4-2.

After the diagnosis of sleep apnea has been made, patients should avoid those things that exacerbate airway obstruction, such as alcohol and CNS depressants (including sleeping pills). Patients with EDS should be cautioned about driving a vehicle or operating machinery. If the patient is overweight, even modestly, weight reduction should be strongly encouraged. The onset of apnea often accompanies a period of rapid weight gain. Subsequent weight loss, if it can be effected, may result in substantial clinical improvement.

If the diagnostic PSG showed that the apneas only occurred while sleeping in a certain position, a modification of sleeping position may be helpful. Reducing nasal or obvious pharyngeal obstruction (e.g., adenotonsillar hypertrophy) can be beneficial.

The tricyclic antidepressant protriptyline, 10–20 mg daily in divided doses, has been useful in patients with mild apnea (13). This agent's action is not totally understood, but it may decrease

TABLE 4-2. Assessment of severity and treatment of sleep apnea

Severity	Apnea plus hypopnea index	Arousals with respiratory events per hour	Lowest O$_2$ saturation	Cardiac effects[a]	Daytime sleepiness	Treatment
Borderline to mild	5–15	<5	90%	Normal	Within normal limits	Weight loss; positional change
Mild to moderate	15–30	5–20	75–90%	Brady-tachycardia associated with respiratory events	Mildly increased sleepiness; MSL 6–11 minutes	Weight loss; positional change; protriptyline, acetazolamide
Moderate to severe	>30	>20	<75%	Frequent PVCs; second-degree A-V block; sinus arrest	Falling asleep while driving or eating; MSL <6 minutes	Nasal CPAP; airway surgery

Note. A-V = atrioventricular; CPAP = continuous positive airway pressure; MSL = mean sleep latency; PVC = premature ventricular contraction.
[a] All cardiac effects must be associated with respiratory events.

the amount of apnea by decreasing the amount of time spent in REM sleep as well as increasing the upper airway muscle tone.

Several recent studies suggest that acetazolamide (Diamox) may play a useful role in the treatment of relatively mild obstructive sleep apnea, in addition to its role in management of central apnea. Thus acetazolamide in doses ranging from 250 mg qd to 250 mg qid might be considered worth a trial in some patients (14, 15).

The use of *continuous positive airway pressure* (CPAP) via a nasal mask has been very successful in the treatment of obstructive apnea (16). While its mode of action is still being debated (acting as a pneumatic splint vs. stimulating nasal receptors), this method has been shown to be very effective in preventing O_2 desaturation, arousals, and arrhythmias, as well as improving daytime alertness. An overnight trial of nasal CPAP in the sleep laboratory is necessary to determine the correct amount of pressure (usually ranging from 5–15 cm H_2O) for each patient. Many patients find CPAP hard to tolerate and awkward to sleep with, leading to compliance rates of only 60–80%.

Intraoral appliances such as several tongue-retaining and mandibular-advancing devices are currently under investigation. However, while often effective, these devices suffer from poor compliance and patient acceptance.

Various surgical procedures have been used to alleviate or bypass the obstruction. A tracheostomy bypasses the upper airway obstruction and is useful in severe life-threatening cases. The uvulopalatopharyngoplasty procedure showed an initial success rate of only 50–70% in cases of apnea, possibly due to poor selection of candidates for the procedure. With improved presurgical evaluation, some centers are reporting success rates as high as 90% (17). Other surgical techniques, including maxillary, mandibular, and hyoid advancement, are being evaluated. Surgical intervention may be the first course of action in children who have sleep apnea caused by excessive lymphoid tissue.

Rapid resolution of some severe cases of obstructive apnea by tracheostomy may produce secondary complications within the family, wherein a chronically ill patient suddenly experiences resolution of symptoms, upsetting the dynamics of family interactional patterns. It may be difficult for families, and the patient, to adjust to a situation in which the patient, who has been identified as chronically ill, and who may not have been able to work or fulfill family responsibilities for some time, is suddenly rendered symptom-free by a surgical procedure. Adjustment can be facilitated by forewarning and appropriate family counseling.

If there is a combination of obstructive and central apneas, the obstructive events should be vigorously treated and often the "central" events will improve. Pure central apnea is rare, often presenting as insomnia rather than EDS. Treatment of central apnea insomnia is discussed further in Chapter 3.

Whatever the treatment chosen, it may be helpful to verify its effectiveness with a repeat PSG study, because patients subjectively tend to overestimate their improvement.

NOCTURNAL HYPOXEMIA

Patients with nocturnal hypoxemia from nonapneic causes (e.g., COPD or cystic fibrosis) often will improve with supplemental oxygen. The correct flow rate should be determined with a supervised overnight study to avoid exacerbating hypoventilation in those patients who are oxygen-sensitive. Patients who tend to hypoventilate during the day often benefit from medroxyprogesterone as a respiratory stimulant (20 mg tid). Routine follow-up PSGs do not appear to contribute significantly to the management of COPD patients (18).

BRONCHOSPASM

Nocturnal symptoms in bronchospastic patients may relate to environmental triggers or the medication schedule. Bedroom exposure to *allergens* can heighten bronchoreactivity in some patients. Other patients who are exposed to allergens in the evening may show a delayed response 6–8 hours later, leading to bronchoconstriction during sleep. These patients can be helped by identification and avoidance of the allergen trigger. Sustained-release theophylline preparations can be given to achieve therapeutic theophylline levels throughout the night. Some patients with severe bronchospasm will have to set an alarm to wake them in order to take inhaled beta-agonist medication midway through the night.

■ OTHER CAUSES OF EXCESSIVE DAYTIME SLEEPINESS

Sleep apnea and narcolepsy are the two leading causes of hypersomnia. However, several less common causes of EDS are outlined below. (For hypersomnolence associated with psychiatric disorders, see Chapter 6.)

SOMNOLENCE ASSOCIATED WITH INSUFFICIENT SLEEP

Individuals who chronically obtain insufficient sleep as a result of occupational, educational, social, or familial demands frequently can become pathologically sleepy. These patients are often unaware that they are voluntarily depriving themselves of sleep, or else they deny this is happening.

The diagnosis of insufficient sleep is suggested when the patient's history and sleep log document chronically short sleep times. Often there will be marked variations in sleep time between weekday and weekend nights. A therapeutic trial of extending sleep time can confirm this diagnosis. Polysomnographic evaluations in these patients demonstrate increased sleep efficiency and increased Stage 3, Stage 4, and REM sleep if patients are permitted to sleep as long as possible. Treatment includes educating patients about their own sleep needs and encouraging consistent extension of their sleep time.

A typical long sleeper may need 9–11 hours of sleep per night, and deprivation below this amount may lead to EDS. If this individual is allowed to get the full amount of sleep, there should be no tendency toward EDS.

IDIOPATHIC CNS HYPERSOMNIA

Idiopathic CNS hypersomnia is a syndrome of persistent daytime somnolence (19). Patients with this disorder note an increasingly irresistible need to sleep during the day that leads to prolonged naps. These naps are lengthy, often 60 minutes or longer, and not very refreshing. When not sleeping, these patients are drowsy and have difficulty concentrating. This excessive sleepiness occurs following normal or even increased amounts of nocturnal sleep. These patients frequently have complaints of "sleep drunkenness" upon awakening.

Patients with idiopathic CNS hypersomnia fall into three categories: (a) Those with a *family history* that is positive for daytime somnolence. In this group there may also be symptoms related to abnormal autonomic function, such as Raynaud's syndrome, orthostatic hypotension, or syncope. (b) Those with a history of *viral infections*, including mononucleosis, viral pneumonia, Guillain-Barré syndrome, and encephalitis. (c) Those without a familial history of EDS or previous significant viral illness, i.e., an *idiopathic group*. These three groups likely differ in terms of etiology and pathophysiology of the hypersomnia syndrome. Some patients with idiopathic hypersomnia are thought to have excessive activity of serotonergic CNS systems, but the evidence for this is still questionable.

LABORATORY FINDINGS

These findings include PSG evidence of normal nocturnal sleep without evidence of breathing disorders, leg jerks, or sleep fragmentation. The MSLT shows a shortened mean sleep latency of about 5–6 minutes.

DIFFERENTIAL DIAGNOSIS

Idiopathic CNS hypersomnia can usually be differentiated from narcolepsy by the absence of cataplexy, hypnagogic hallucinations, and sleep paralysis. Sleep apnea is suggested by a history of snoring. A PSG and MSLT are necessary to differentiate idiopathic CNS hypersomnia from the other causes of EDS.

TREATMENT

Treatment of this hypersomnia is difficult. Various medications, including the serotonin antagonist methysergide, as well as scheduled naps, have been tried with minimal success. Stimulant medication may be useful, but the majority of patients still complain of daytime sleepiness and take daily naps.

KLEINE-LEVIN SYNDROME

This syndrome is a periodic hypersomnia, usually occurring in males, and commonly beginning in the patient's teens (20). Typically, the patient will have one or more episodes yearly, characterized by periods of excessive sleepiness often lasting weeks. During these hypersomnolent times, the patient can be aroused, but when awake he or she is confused and agitated, and shows a loss of sexual inhibitions. While in this somnolent state patients can demonstrate insatiable appetites, especially if presented with food. After the episode clears, the patient has minimal recollection of the hypersomnolent period. Between attacks the patient eats, sleeps, and mentates in a normal fashion. Usually this disorder spontaneously remits by age 40. The etiology of Kleine-Levin syndrome is unknown, but disorders of several brain regions, including the thalamus, brain stem, frontal lobes, and hypothalamus (21), have been suggested.

DIFFERENTIAL DIAGNOSIS

The periodic nature of the somnolence, along with the abnormal behavior, confusion, and compulsive eating, differentiates Kleine-Levin syndrome from other common causes of excessive somnolence. Other psychiatric disorders (especially manic depressive disorder and schizophrenia), drug-induced states, and metabolic and inflammatory disorders should be considered.

LABORATORY FINDINGS

EEG evaluations done during the wakeful portions of a hypersomnolent episode have shown mild intermittent slowing. Nocturnal sleep has been reported to lack Stage 3 and Stage 4. There have also been reports of shortened REM latency and even of an occasional sleep onset REM period being recorded. Although analysis of cerebrospinal fluid is usually normal in these patients, there have been reports of elevated levels of 5-hydroxyindoleacetic acid in a few cases.

TREATMENT

Because this condition is self-limited, many patients are not treated. Stimulant medication has been useful to treat the somnolence but can worsen the behavioral problems. Lithium has met with some success in prophylaxis of the hypersomnolent episodes.

MENSTRUATION-ASSOCIATED HYPERSOMNIA

Some women become periodically hypersomnolent around the time of their menses. They often exhibit abnormal behavior (e..g., withdrawal, apathy, irritability) during these somnolent times and may awaken only for bathroom visits. After their menses pass, these women resume their normal behavior and daytime alertness. The etiology is not known, but hypothalamic dysfunction is hypothesized (22).

LABORATORY FINDINGS

Decreased amounts of Stage 3 and Stage 4 sleep have been noted in the few cases of this uncommon disorder that were polygraphically evaluated.

DIFFERENTIAL DIAGNOSIS

The characteristic relationship of the hypersomnia with the menstrual cycle differentiates this disorder from most other causes of EDS. A careful history regarding medications used for menstrual symptoms must be obtained to exclude medication-induced somnolence.

TREATMENT

There have been reports of total cessation of the hypersomnia when ovulation was blocked by oral contraceptive agents.

HYPERSOMNIA ASSOCIATED WITH DRUGS AND ALCOHOL

Patients in this category fall into two general groups: (a) those that are somnolent due to the direct sedating effect of a drug; or (b) those that are somnolent as a result of drug withdrawal.

a. Patients who chronically take *stimulants* (amphetamine, methylphenidate, caffeine) for mood elevation, fatigue, and as a treatment of EDS from any cause, can become tolerant to those substances. As tolerance develops, these patients are frequently in a state of withdrawal, characterized by excessive sleepiness, lassitude, difficulty waking in the morning, depression, and increased appetite. This withdrawal due to tolerance leads to an escalation in stimulant dose and ultimately a withdrawal of even greater severity.

These patients must be differentiated from patients with EDS of a psychiatric etiology. Patients who take stimulants chronically can be diagnostically challenging in that they frequently initiated the stimulant as treatment for an undiagnosed hypersomnia. It is useful to withdraw them from the stimulant for a few weeks and reassess their symptoms. If they are still somnolent, a nocturnal PSG, MSLT, and confirmatory drug screen should be obtained to evaluate for other causes of EDS. A PSG should be obtained after a drug-free interval of 14 days, because patients who are acutely withdrawing from stimulants can exhibit short sleep latencies and excessive amounts of REM sleep (i.e., REM rebound).

b. Individuals who chronically use *CNS depressants* (barbiturates, opiates, benzodiazepines, tricyclic antidepressants, major tranquilizers, beta blockers, and alcohol) for medical reasons or as a self-treatment in response to anxiety can develop daytime somnolence. Many patients (especially the elderly) may be trying to treat a coexistent insomnia and have significant drug carryover the following day. A good history of the patient's medication use usually makes the condition apparent. The patient should be reevaluated after suspect medications are withdrawn.

EXCESSIVE DAYTIME SLEEPINESS ASSOCIATED WITH NOCTURNAL MYOCLONUS

Patients with PLMS usually complain of insomnia (see Chapter 3) but can have EDS as a symptom as well. It is felt that sleep fragmentation due to repetitive arousals associated with leg jerks is the mechanism producing daytime sleepiness. Nocturnal myoclonus is often unsuspected by the patient, and a polysomnographic evaluation is required for diagnosis. Nocturnal myoclonus can coexist with either narcolepsy or sleep apnea.

LABORATORY FINDINGS

Evidence of PLMS is found on a PSG. Total sleep time, sleep efficiency, and Stage 3 and Stage 4 sleep often decrease, while Stage 1 and Stage 2 sleep increases.

TREATMENT

Patients whose somnolence is attributed to arousals associated with leg jerks have been treated with clonazepam (1–3 mg) or temazepam (15–30 mg) prior to bedtime. These medications decrease the number of arousals while having no effect on the number of leg jerks present.

■ REFERENCES

1. Hoddes E, Zarcone V, Smythe H, et al: Quantification of sleepiness: a new approach. Psychophysiology 10:431–436, 1973
2. Parkes JD: The sleepy driver, in Driving and Epilepsy and Other Causes of Impaired Consciousness. Edited by Godwin-Austen RB, Espir MLE. London, Royal Society of Medicine, 1983
3. Mosko SS, Shampain DS, Sassinn SF: Nocturnal REM latency and sleep disturbance in narcolepsy. Sleep 7:115–125, 1984
4. Bixler E, Kales A, Soldatos C, et al: Prevalence of sleep disorders: a survey of the Los Angeles metropolitan area. Am J Psychiatry 136:1257–1262, 1979
5. Mignot E, Guilleminault C, Bowersox S, et al: Role of central alpha-1 adrenoceptors in canine narcolepsy. J Clin Invest 82:885–894, 1988
6. Langdon N, Lock C, Welsh K, et al: Immune factors in narcolepsy. Sleep 9:143–148, 1986
7. Inoko H, Ando A, Tseuji K, et al: HLA-DQ chain DNA restriction fragments can differentiate between healthy and narcoleptic individuals with HLA-DR2. Immunogenetics 23:126–128, 1986
8. Mitler MM, Shafor R, Hajdukovich R, et al: Treatment of narcolepsy: objective studies on methylphenidate, pemoline, and protriptyline. Sleep 9:260–264, 1986
9. Guilleminault C: Obstructive sleep apnea syndrome: a review. Psychiatr Clin North Am 10:607–621, 1987
10. Williams AJ, Houston D, Finberg S, et al: Sleep apnea syndrome and essential hypertension. Am J Cardiol 55:1019–1022, 1985
11. Flenley DC: Sleep in chronic obstructive lung disease. Clin Chest Med 6:651–661, 1985
12. Douglas NA: Asthma at night. Clin Chest Med 5:663–674, 1985

13. Lombard R, Zwillich C: Medical therapy of obstructive sleep apnea. Med Clin North Am 69:1317–1335, 1985
14. Tojima H, Kunitomo F, Kimura H, et al: Effects of acetazolamide in patients with the sleep apnea syndrome. Thorax 43:113–119, 1988
15. Whyte KF, Gould GA, Airlie MA: Role of protriptyline and acetazolamide in the sleep apnea/hypopnea syndrome. Sleep 11:463–472, 1988
16. Sullivan C, Issa FG, Berthon-Jones M, et al: Reversal of obstructive sleep apnea by continuous positive airway pressure applied through the nares. Lancet, April 18, 1981, pp 862–865
17. Riley R, Powell N, Guilleminault C: Current surgical concepts for treating obstructive sleep apnea syndrome. J Oral Maxillofac Surg 45:149–157, 1986
18. Connaugh JJ, Catteral JR, Elton RA, et al: Do sleep studies contribute to the management of patients with severe chronic obstructive pulmonary disease. Am Rev Respir Dis 138:341–344, 1988
19. Guilleminault C: Disorders of excessive sleepiness. Ann Clin Res 17:209–219, 1985
20. Orlosky M: The Kleine-Levin syndrome: a review. Psychosomatics 23:609–617, 1982
21. Gadoth N, Dickerman Z, Bechar M, et al: Episodic hormone secretion during sleep in Kleine-Levin syndrome: evidence for hypothalamic dysfunction. Brain Dev 9:309–315, 1987
22. Billiard M, Guilleminault C, Dement W: A menstruation-linked periodic hypersomnia. Neurology 25:436–443, 1975

■ ADDITIONAL READINGS

Martin RJ: Cardiorespiratory Disorders During Sleep. Mount Kisco, NY, Futura Publishing Co, 1984

Roth B: Narcolepsy and Hypersomnia. Basel, S Karger, 1980

5 PARASOMNIAS

Parasomnias, or events around sleep, are a group of disturbances of sleep that range from extremely common to very rare. They occur more frequently in children and are generally benign in nature. Although some require specific treatment, the majority of them seem to precipitate worry in the patient or family that can be relieved by adequate explanation and understanding of the unusual event. The four general categories of parasomnias discussed here are (a) parasomnias associated with REM sleep (e.g., nightmares); (b) arousal disorders (including sleepwalking and night terrors); (c) sleep/wake transition disorders; and (d) miscellaneous parasomnias.

■ PARASOMNIAS ASSOCIATED WITH REM SLEEP

NIGHTMARES

Nightmares are long and frightening dreams arising from REM sleep. They tend to be most common in children, although 30–50% of adults remember an occasional nightmare, perhaps on the order of one per year. Stress increases the frequency of nightmares. A severely traumatic event may be followed by frequent nightmares in which the event is relived, which in turn may be a component of a posttraumatic stress disorder (PTSD) (see below). A sudden increase in nightmares in a young adult might be a sign of an impending schizophrenic break. Early stress (e.g., child abuse) does not appear to result in increased incidence of nightmares later in life; but there are adults suffering from frequent nightmares who Hartmann (1) characterizes as vulnerable, open, and sensitive persons with thin boundaries.

SLEEP PARALYSIS

Sleep paralysis can occur independently of narcolepsy, and will present clinically as partial or complete paralysis occurring at the onset of awakening from sleep, most probably accompanying REM periods. In addition to its relationship with narcolepsy (as described in Chapter 4), sleep paralysis can occur (a) as an isolated episode in non-narcoleptic people; (b) as a rare familial disorder unaccompanied by other symptoms, with a number of family members having a similar complaint; and (c) in association with other hypersomnolence disorders such as obstructive sleep apnea. If treatment is deemed necessary, one should begin with a low-dose tricyclic, such as 10 mg desipramine or imipramine, and gradually increase the dosage until the symptoms are blocked. Response will usually occur within 1–2 days after reaching adequate dosage. Other drugs associated with REM suppression may not eliminate the paralysis.

REM SLEEP BEHAVIOR DISORDER

REM sleep behavior disorder is a parasomnia characterized by the emergence of complex and vigorous behaviors during REM sleep (2). Punching, kicking, and leaping from the bed in an apparent attempt to enact dreams are typically seen and can be a cause of serious physical injury. The syndrome has been described predominantly in males in their 60s and 70s. The syndrome may result from damage to the brain systems controlling the normal muscle atonia of REM sleep, and a number of cases have been associated with neurological conditions such as dementia, hemorrhage, or degeneration. Nocturnal polysomnograms (PSGs) tend to show high REM density, increased slow wave sleep, and an increased number of limb movements in non-REM sleep. Differential diagnosis includes other parasomnia disorders as well as seizure disorders.

Treatment of REM sleep behavior disorder with clonazepam has been effective in most cases. Because most patients with this disorder are elderly, a conservative approach would be to start clonazepam at 0.25 mg hs and gradually increase the dose until control is effected. If excessive daytime sedation occurs, one should consider switching to desipramine, beginning at 10 mg and again increasing the dose until the nocturnal behavior disorder is suppressed.

SLEEP-RELATED IMPAIRED PENILE ERECTIONS

Sleep-related impaired penile erections are usually detected during a laboratory study of nocturnal penile tumescence, most often undertaken in the evaluation of male impotence. Laboratory evidence of impaired penile erections is most often an indication of an underlying organic factor, as psychological factors infrequently (but occasionally) impair nocturnal penile tumescence. Among the organic factors known to cause both impaired nocturnal penile tumescence and impotence are diabetes mellitus, endocrine disorders, hyperprolactinemia, penile diseases (including priapism and Peyronie's disease), disorders of the central and autonomic nervous system, respiratory and hematological disorders, polycythemia, lymphoma, alcoholism, psychotropic and adrenergic blocking drugs, penile arterial insufficiency, and penile venous pathology. Diagnosis requires full medical evaluation, and treatment is directed toward correcting the underlying cause of the impaired erections.

SLEEP-RELATED PAINFUL ERECTIONS

Sleep-related painful erections constitute a rare disorder where the patient awakens several times during the night with very painful erections, which, after the patient awakens, may slowly disappear over minutes, along with the associated pain. Although waking sexual function is usually unimpaired, serious cases result in insomnia. The patient should be evaluated for underlying penile pathology, including phimosis or Peyronie's disease, which should be treated as appropriate. This parasomnia often does not require treatment, although in severe cases the associated insomnia may be treated with an REM-suppressant drug.

REM SLEEP-RELATED SINUS ARREST

REM sleep-related sinus arrest is a rare condition that has been reported in individuals without any other apparent cardiac abnormalities, and with only vague cardiac-related symptoms (3). These patients may experience prolonged periods of asystole, up to 9 seconds in duration, which occur primarily during REM sleep. Patients diagnosed as having this abnormality will require close cardiac follow-up and consideration for possible pacemaker implantation.

■ SLEEPWALKING AND NIGHT TERRORS

PRESENTING COMPLAINTS

- Nocturnal confusional or walking episodes while still apparently asleep
- Unusual or bizarre nocturnal behavioral episodes
- Sitting up in bed, crying or screaming inconsolably, accompanied by fast heart rate and rapid breathing

CLINICAL CHARACTERISTICS

Sleepwalking and night terrors are related parasomnias that occur more often in children than in adults. These parasomnias are characterized by motor or autonomic activity during a state of partial arousal from sleep, sometimes called "half-sleep."

In children, the majority of sleepwalkers will not even leave the bed, but rather make repetitive movements while sitting up on the edge of the bed. When these children do leave the bed, they will tend to walk around the house with their eyes open, avoiding bumping into familiar objects. Behaviors tend to be quite simple in nature, and there is minimal talking. Vocalization during more disturbed episodes may include cries for help, yelling about trying to escape, and possibly shouting out someone's name. If sleepwalkers are spoken to, they will usually not respond, and will avoid eye contact. If awakened, there will usually be a period of disorientation lasting several minutes. Most sleepwalkers will return to their bed in time, and one appropriate way of dealing with them is to try to calmly usher them back in the direction of their bedroom. Recall of these events is usually poor or lacking, and dream reports are more likely to have vague static and sometimes fearful images rather than the typical story lines seen in REM dreams. The sleepwalking episodes can last anywhere from a few seconds to a few minutes, with the average episode being about 6 minutes. Episodes up to 1 hour in duration have been reported in the literature.

Sleepwalking and night terror episodes can be quite dangerous (4), and approximately 75% of all sleepwalkers and night terror sufferers have reported actual injuries or the potential for injuries during their episodes. One study indicated that greater than 50% of all sleepwalkers had reported leaving the house during an episode at one time or another. Some sleepwalkers can be quite combative upon sudden awakening. Some studies have found that 28% of sleepwalkers and 55% of those suffering from night terrors have reported violent behavior during these arousal episodes (5, 6).

Night terrors represent a more severe nocturnal arousal. Similar to sleepwalking, they occur during the first 3 hours of the night when Stage 3 and Stage 4 sleep predominates. These episodes tend to begin with a loud cry and the onset of a prolonged period of apparent intense anxiety, with evidence of tachycardia, increased blood pressure, dilated pupils, and sweating. The typical episode lasts in the range of 6 minutes, and there can be a significant additional period of confusion after the episode (7). Attempts to arouse someone amid a night terror are probably ill-advised, because disorientation may continue up to 30 minutes after arousal from the episode. The episodes are more common in deep sleepers and in males, and are most frequently not remembered the next morning (in marked contrast to REM nightmares).

Although sleepwalking and night terror activity can look distinctly different, it is not uncommon for elements of the night terror and the sleepwalking to occur together in the same arousal episode. One study has shown that 55% of adult sleepwalkers also suffer from night terrors, and 72% of night terror sufferers also complain of sleepwalking (5, 6). It has been postulated that these parasomnias represent the same disorder of arousal displaying a continuum of severity, with sleepwalking being the milder form and night terrors being the more severe form of arousal.

There is evidence for three major classifications of sleepwalking and night terror sufferers:

1. Childhood sleepwalking and night terrors, with an age of onset in the range of 4–6 years, usually terminating by adolescence.

2. Young adult familial sleepwalking and night terrors, with a strong family history of nocturnal arousal disorders beginning early in childhood and extending into early adulthood without remission. This group may exhibit a lesser degree or no evidence of psychopathology.
3. Adult sleepwalking and night terrors. This group tends to have a later onset of symptomatology, beginning around age 10 with early childhood sleepwalking and night terrors, interrupted by many years of being asymptomatic and then recurring after particular stresses. Individuals in this group exhibit a greater degree of psychopathology.

It is important to note that the initial complaint may be voiced by parents or bed partners, since the patients are usually unaware of most of the behaviors accompanying these disorders.

INCIDENCE

It has been estimated that approximately 15% of all children aged 5–12 will sleepwalk at least once, and that 3–6% will sleepwalk more than once (8). Childhood somnambulists usually grow out of the condition by adolescence. Less than half of 1% of adults walk in their sleep. It is estimated that 10–20% of all sleepwalkers have family members who have also walked in their sleep, and there is evidence that relatives of sleepwalkers tend to have deeper than normal sleep (9). The incidence of night terrors appears to be less than that for sleepwalking in all age groups.

PATHOPHYSIOLOGY AND ETIOLOGY

Sleepwalking and night terrors are disorders of arousal from slow wave or Stage 3 and Stage 4 of non-REM sleep, possibly reflecting an impairment (developmental or other) in the normal mechanisms of arousal from deep sleep, resulting in partial arousals in which motor behaviors are activated but full consciousness does not return. This may be one reason why parasomnias are more common in the "immature" nervous system of children, and why children typically grow out of them in time.

Many patients with sleepwalking or night terrors have a

family history of the disorder, suggesting a genetic component. In children, night terrors not infrequently begin in the several months following an illness with a high fever.

About half of all patients report having major stressful life events occurring before the onset of their disorder. Most also indicate that stress increases the frequency of their episodes, as do fatigue, changes in sleep environment, anxiety, fevers, loss of sleep, or use of various medications such as lithium, neuroleptics, or hypnotics. Neuroleptic medications may precipitate sleepwalking in adults who have had no previous episodes.

Adult patients with early onset and a strong familial tendency may have a somewhat different course in treatment than those who have had the onset later in childhood and who exhibit a greater degree of psychopathology. A great number of adult sleepwalkers and night terror sufferers will have had long stretches of time without any episodes and then will have a reoccurrence after a major psychological stress or trauma. Kales et al. (5) examined Minnesota Multiphasic Personality Inventory (MMPI) profiles of sleep walkers and night terror sufferers and found that these individuals had difficulty with appropriate expression of aggression and often had a strong tendency toward internalization of emotions. We have found night terror sufferers to have a greater than expected incidence of alcoholism within the family as well as other traumatic events occurring during childhood. There also seems to be an increased incidence of depressive episodes in the background of adult night terror sufferers.

LABORATORY FINDINGS

Nocturnal PSG recordings during somnambulistic or night terror episodes typically show these episodes to emerge from Stage 3 or Stage 4 sleep, with fairly normal sleep prior to the sudden appearance of the parasomnia event. Nothing else in the sleep recording is diagnostic of parasomnia disorders, and this fact, combined with the fact that these events tend to be rare and usually difficult to reproduce in the laboratory environment, makes routine PSG recordings of little value in diagnosis. Of course, if a typical event is recorded under laboratory conditions, especially if it includes a videotape of the behaviors, the diagnosis is clear.

DIFFERENTIAL DIAGNOSIS

1. *Nightmares* tend to occur in REM sleep usually in the middle of the night or in the morning when REM sleep is more prevalent. Because REM sleep is a time of muscle paralysis, nightmares are not associated with movement during the actual dream. There tends to be good recall of the dream afterward, and the dreamer is very quickly alert after awakening. There can be a significant amount of anxiety, accompanied by an increase in pulse rate, but the patient usually can be easily calmed. Nightmares can occur during drug or alcohol withdrawal. They also may accompany depression or the use of beta blockers, and are as well a common element of a PTSD.
2. *Automatic behavior and dissociative states* are usually found in adults with disturbed psychiatric backgrounds. Often such events will be seen to occur during waking as well as in sleep. Behavior may be much more complex than is seen in a typical sleepwalking or night terror episode. Episodes involving automatic behavior and dissociative states can last for several hours, and the sufferer frequently will not return to his or her own bed.
3. *Sleep drunkenness or confusional arousals* are states of partial awakening when an individual is extremely fatigued, or affected by sedatives or alcohol. They are also seen as part of the narcolepsy syndrome. Although aggressive behavior is common during these states, there is no good evidence that a purposefully criminal act can occur during such episodes.
4. *Psychomotor epileptic seizures* tend to be short in duration, and no response can be elicited from the patient during the episodes. An EEG may be necessary to distinguish these episodes from sleepwalking or night terrors. The EEG should follow a night of partial sleep deprivation and should include an adequate sleep recording.
5. *Panic attacks* may be confused with parasomnias. It is not uncommon for patients with nocturnal panic attacks to present

with episodes of tachycardia, shortness of breath, sweating, and extreme fear or terror. The main distinction between the panic attack and the night terror is that the patient will be alert and aware of surroundings during the panic attack and will have very clear recall of the onset and the events around the episode the next morning.
6. *REM sleep behavior disorder* (discussed earlier in this chapter) may be confused with night terrors, although sudden onset in elderly patients, characteristic of REM sleep behavior disorder, is not characteristic of night terrors.

It is usually unnecessary to do any specific laboratory studies for diagnosis of sleepwalking and night terrors. In persistent cases, especially those in which there may be some concern about possible psychomotor epilepsy, an EEG may be indicated. If there is still confusion or concern about persistent and frequent problems, a PSG could be obtained to clarify whether the episodes indeed are occurring early in the night from Stage 3 or Stage 4 sleep. This could also provide information as to whether there may be EEG abnormalities during nocturnal sleep that were not seen on a routine EEG.

TREATMENT

Treatment of sleepwalking and night terrors is dependent upon the type of clinical presentation:

1. Most *children with night terrors or somnambulism* will grow out of the symptoms with increasing physiological maturity. Reassurance of parents and the child is indicated. Sleepwalkers should be protected by appropriate locks on the doors and windows to preclude the patient's leaving the house and being put in a dangerous position. Inexpensive ultrasonic burglar alarms can be used to alert others in the house that the patient has started walking. It is often advantageous to allow the sleepwalker to sleep on the first floor to avoid the risk of falling out a window. In severe cases one should explore the possibility of psychotherapy, as well as a low dose of a tricyclic (e.g., desipramine 10–15 mg) or a benzodiazepine (e.g., triazolam

0.125 mg or diazepam 2 mg hs), which may decrease the frequency of the events either by suppressing arousal or suppressing deep Stage 3 and Stage 4 sleep. In children with frequent and severe night terrors, 10–50 mg imipramine or desipramine might be given for a period of approximately 6 weeks. After discontinuation of the drug, many of these children remain symptom-free.

2. *Young adults with familial night terrors* should be evaluated for possible psychotherapy, emphasizing exploration for evidence of stressful early childhood events or recent events. Low-dose benzodiazepines or low-dose tricyclics can be tried, although our general experience with this group of young adults suggests that they do not respond well to medication or psychotherapy, and successful treatment may be difficult.

3. *Adult sleepwalking and night terrors* are frequently amenable to psychotherapeutic intervention. We have seen several cases in which short-term exploratory and insight-oriented therapy, including aiding the patient to express emotions more directly, has resulted in alleviation of night terror and sleepwalking symptoms within a matter of weeks. For those suffering from potentially dangerous sleepwalking and night terror episodes, it is most appropriate to consider medication early on, in conjunction with psychotherapy. We frequently begin with desipramine 10 mg hs and gradually increase the dose until the episodes are significantly diminished. Imipramine and nortriptyline have also been used successfully. Although most of the patients respond to a relatively low dose (between 10 and 50 mg) of these drugs, there are a number of cases that have evidence of concurrent depression and that require full antidepressant dosages. After resolution of symptoms, the patient should be encouraged to stay in treatment until there is an adequate resolution of conflicts, at which time the medication should be slowly tapered as tolerated.

■ OTHER PARASOMNIAS

A variety of other unusual nocturnal symptoms are classified as parasomnias, or events around sleep. The most frequently occurring are briefly described below.

RHYTHMIC MOVEMENT DISORDER

Rhythmic movement disorder, also called "head-banging" or *jactatio capitis nocturnus*, is a disorder of early childhood that usually disappears by adolescence. Rhythmic movement of the head, and at times whole body rocking, will generally occur just before onset of sleep and continue during light sleep. The rocking movement usually disappears by the time the child is in slow wave sleep, and there is no evidence of daytime behavioral problems. Although there are many organic and psychological theories as to its cause, none are satisfactory. There are no effective treatments at this time. Benzodiazepines may suppress the movements for a period of time, but these agents tend to lose effectiveness after several weeks.

SLEEP STARTS

Sleep starts include hypnic jerks and sensory starts. A *hypnic jerk* is a generalized body jerk that occurs at the onset of sleep. Hypnic jerks are almost universal, nonpathological, and probably a minor arousal response to some subtle stimulus at the time of sleep onset. *Sensory starts* include sensory experiences, often of a dream-like nature, that can accompany a hypnic jerk, or occur by themselves, at the time of sleep onset, and can arouse one back into wakefulness. Sensory starts are benign. Both forms of sleep starts should be treated with reassurance of their normality.

SLEEPTALKING

Sleeptalking is a common event, most often occurring during Stage 1 or Stage 2 sleep. It often occurs when an individual who is just dropping off to sleep is addressed with a question. There will often be no recall of what has been said. Extreme tiredness may make sleeptalking more likely. Sleeptalking does not seem to be closely associated with other arousal disorders such as sleepwalking or night terrors. Some cases are severe enough, with talking throughout the night, to cause a significant disruption to the sleep of the bed partner. Milder cases should be reassured; however, no specific treatments can be recommended for more severe cases at this time. Sleeptalking is generally unresponsive to medication or psychotherapy.

HYPNAGOGIC HALLUCINATIONS

Hypnagogic hallucinations have been described in Chapter 4 in terms of their association with narcolepsy. These hallucinations can also occur in nonnarcoleptic individuals, and at times the experience is very terrifying. Occurrences are sporadic in nature and tend to accompany periods of sleep disruption, increased stress, or depression. A typical hypnagogic hallucination is experienced as lying in bed awake, suddenly feeling unable to move (sleep paralysis), and then being besieged by disturbing auditory or visual hallucinatory experiences. Occasionally, a partial paralysis of respiratory muscles results in a sensation of imminent death, requiring the patient to strongly resist and force himself or herself back to full awareness. These events can be strikingly dramatic, inducing an intense preoccupation with the abnormal events as well as the content of the hallucinatory experiences. The events typically occur in Stage 1 and Stage 2 non-REM sleep.

In general, no treatment is necessary. In time, many patients will begin to realize there are no particular dangers, and they may actually begin to enjoy the experiences. Like the sleep paralysis that often accompanies them, hypnagogic hallucinations are responsive to low-dose tricyclics if treatment is deemed necessary.

SLEEP BRUXISM

Sleep bruxism is a very common disorder consisting of tooth grinding during sleep. Bruxism probably occurs in 5–10% of all children and declines in frequency with age. No cause is known, but bruxism is at times exacerbated by anxiety. It occurs mainly in Stage 2 sleep, and there is evidence of increased amplitude of EMG activity in the masseter and the temporalis muscles. The treatment of choice is a dental device to avoid wearing down the teeth. Other treatments that have shown some success include muscle relaxation exercises, hypnotic medication, biofeedback, hypnosis, and occlusal adjustment.

SLEEP-RELATED ABNORMAL SWALLOWING SYNDROME

Sleep-related abnormal swallowing syndrome is characterized by complaints of choking on pooled saliva that has not been swallowed during sleep. There is no clear treatment for the disorder, but patients should be evaluated for the presence of a pharyngeal pouch.

NOCTURNAL PAROXYSMAL DYSTONIA

Nocturnal paroxysmal dystonia is a rare syndrome of coarse, often violent movements of the limbs occurring during non-REM sleep and having no associated EEG abnormality. These movements seem to be triggered by an arousal. Cases reported to date appear to respond well to carbamazepine (15 mg/kg daily) (10).

SLEEP-RELATED TONIC SPASMS

Sleep-related tonic spasms, or proctalgia fugax, are intense spasms of the levator ani muscle that can cause excruciating pain. The pain is usually felt in the rectum just above the anus and can last from a few seconds to a half an hour. There is as yet no known organic cause. The syndrome may have some relationship to anxiety. It is known to occur occasionally during the daytime as well as at night. There is no effective treatment other than reassurance that it will not progress or lead to more serious problems.

SUDDEN UNEXPLAINED NOCTURNAL DEATH SYNDROME

Sudden unexplained nocturnal death syndrome, also known as "Bangungut" in the Philippines, "Non-laitai" in Laos, and "Pokkuri" in Japan (11), is a syndrome of unexpected nocturnal deaths occurring in young Asian males. Cardiac conduction defects have been found in postmortem analysis in many of the victims, and there is evidence that many victims also suffered from night terrors, suggesting a relationship between the autonomic arousal associated with night terrors and the cardiac conduction abnormalities leading to nocturnal death.

BENIGN NEONATAL SLEEP MYOCLONUS

Benign neonatal sleep myoclonus is a rare syndrome of rhythmic jerking of hands, arms, and legs, as well as occasional repetitive jerking of fingers, wrists, elbows, and ankles, that occurs in early infancy. The movements may occur at sleep onset and later on in sleep as well. Symptoms tend to disappear by ages 1–2. It is a benign condition that can be diagnosed by the presence of a normal EEG as well as the fact that it occurs only during sleep.

This syndrome is thought to represent a developmental abnormality in the reticular activating system, possibly related to sleep starts, that resolves with maturation of the nervous system.

PRIMARY SNORING

Primary snoring is sometimes considered to be a parasomnia. As discussed earlier (see Chapter 4), primary snoring may be symptomatic of a sleep-related breathing disorder. When found in the absence of a breathing disorder, it may still be a distressing symptom, leading to considerable family sleep disruption, or the disruption of sleep in nearby persons. If snoring is positional (e.g., worse while sleeping on the back), a simple remedy such as putting pajama tops on backward and placing a tennis ball in a front pocket (to discourage sleeping on the back) may suffice. Very severe cases may require surgical intervention, and the palatopharyngoplasty procedure may provide substantial benefit (12).

■ REFERENCES

1. Hartmann E: The Nightmare. New York, Basic Books, 1984
2. Schenk CH, Bundie SR, Patterson AC, et al: Rapid eye movement sleep behavior disorder. A treatable parasomnia. JAMA 257:1786–1789, 1987
3. Guilleminault C, Pool P, Motta J, et al: Sinus arrest during REM sleep in young adults. N Engl J Med 311:1006–1010, 1985
4. Hartmann E: Two case reports: night terrors with sleep-walking—a potentially lethal disorder. J Nerv Ment Dis 171:503–505, 1983
5. Kales JD, Kales A, Soldatos CR, et al: Night terrors: clinical characteristics and personality patterns. Arch Gen Psychiatry 37:1413–1417, 1980
6. Kales A, Soldatos CR, Caldwell AB, et al: Somnambulism: clinical characteristics and personality patterns. Arch Gen Psychiatry 37:1406–1410, 1980
7. Fisher C, Kahn E, Edwards A, et al: A psychophysiological study of nightmares, and night terrors. Physiological aspects of the stage 4 night terror. J Nerv Ment Dis 157:75–98, 1973
8. Bakwin H: Sleep-walking in twins. Lancet, August 29, 1970, pp 446–447
9. Davies E, Hayes M, Kirman BH: Somnambulism. Lancet 1:186, 1942

10. Lee BI, Lesser RP, Pippenger CE, et al: Familial paroxysmal hypnogenic dystonia. Sleep 9:54–60, 1986
11. Melles RB, Katz B: Night terrors and sudden unexplained nocturnal death. Med Hypotheses 26:149–154, 1988
12. Rice D, Persky M: Snoring: clinical implications and its treatment. Otolaryngol Head Neck Surg 95:28–30, 1986

6 MEDICAL AND PSYCHIATRIC DISORDERS AND SLEEP

■ MEDICAL DISORDERS AND SLEEP

Sleep can be disrupted by the *symptoms* associated with medical illnesses (e.g., insomnia due to pain from any cause). Medical conditions can also affect sleep *directly*, as is seen with hypersomnia associated with hydrocephalus or neoplasms of the CNS. In such conditions, the sleep complaint tends to wax and wane along with the severity of the medical illness. If the sleep abnormality persists once the underlying medical condition improves, other factors (e.g., psychophysiological insomnia) may have become involved.

SYMPTOMS OF MEDICAL DISORDERS DISRUPTIVE TO SLEEP

Frequent symptoms that may accompany a large variety of medical disorders, and that may significantly disrupt sleep, include abnormal movements from any cause, diarrhea, night sweats, nocturia, nocturnal confusion, pain from any cause, palpitations, pruritus, and respiratory symptoms.

SPECIFIC MEDICAL CONDITIONS ASSOCIATED WITH DISORDERED SLEEP

CNS neoplasms can cause movement disorders and seizures leading to insomnia. Midline lesions (in the pineal gland, hypothalamus, third ventricle, or brain stem) often lead to increased intracranial pressure. Patients with these lesions may demonstrate an increased sleepiness, ranging from mildly increased daytime somnolence to obtundation. Patients with subdural hematomas, multiple sclerosis, neurosyphilis, trypanosomiasis, or head trauma, or those who are postencephalitic, frequently exhibit excessive daytime sleepiness (EDS).

Parkinson's disease patients frequently have disturbed sleep with a prolonged sleep latency and an increase in time awake after sleep onset. Although the characteristic tremor disappears during sleep, it can return during many of the frequent arousals (1). The abnormal movements characteristic of degenerative diseases of the basal ganglia typically disappear during sleep.

Endocrinopathies are notorious for disrupting sleep. Hypothyroid patients frequently complain of fatigue and sleepiness, and demonstrate a decrease in Stage 3 and Stage 4 sleep that normalizes with thyroid hormone supplementation (2). Hypothyroid infants show a decreased amount of sleep spindle activity, with this activity increasing after hormone therapy. Hyperthyroid patients have increased Stage 3 and Stage 4 sleep before treatment. Addison's disease and Cushing's syndrome have both been associated with insomnia. Patients with Cushing's syndrome tend to have decreased amounts of slow wave sleep, whereas those with Addison's disease have increased amounts of Stage 3 and Stage 4 sleep.

Diabetic individuals can have poor sleep for a variety of reasons. Nocturnal hypoglycemia (Somogyi effect), nocturnal diarrhea, and pain from peripheral neuropathies all can disrupt sleep.

Primary respiratory disorders such as chronic obstructive pulmonary disease, cystic fibrosis, and asthma may have significant sleep pathology and associated complaints. These disorders are considered in more detail in Chapter 4.

Fibrositis, or *fibromyalgia*, is a common disorder characterized by chronic fatigue, muscular aches, and nonrestorative sleep. Physical examination is notable for characteristic "trigger points," including tender areas in the trapezius, the medial fat pad of knee, the iliac crest, the lateral epicondyle, and others. Patients with fibrositis frequently complain of "nonrestorative" sleep—that is, they may sleep for a normal period of time but awaken feeling tired, unrefreshed, or "nonrestored." Such patients frequently have an increased amount of alpha frequency activity in their slow wave sleep EEG recordings, termed an "alpha-delta"-type sleep pattern (see Figure 6-1). Moldofsky suggests that this syndrome represents a physiological arousal disorder (3). Alpha-delta sleep patterns can be seen in other disorders, including sedative-hypnotic-related insomnias.

Epstein-Barr virus (EBV) often includes sleep complaints such as insomnia and nonrestorative sleep. Polysomnographic studies demonstrate frequent abnormalities in patients with EBV. These abnormalities are of varying types, including alpha-delta patterns.

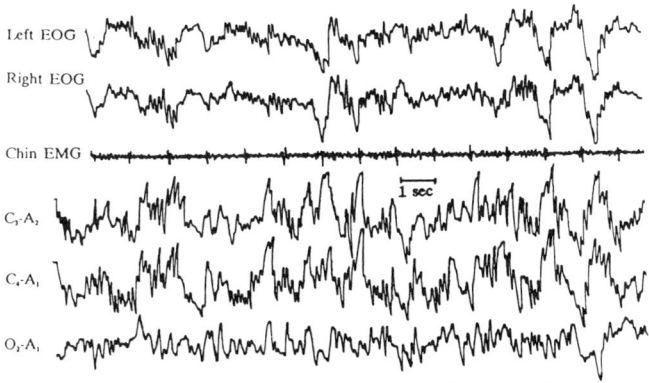

FIGURE 6-1. **Excessive alpha-frequency activity superimposed upon a basically delta slow wave sleep background.**

This illustration was taken from the PSG record of a 41-year-old female with sleep complaints of both insomnia and EDS, and a possible EBV syndrome. This patient was taking alprazolam 1 mg qd and trazodone 150 mg qd.

Arthritis may be associated with poor sleep, including frequent arousals and an increase in alpha frequency activity in the sleep EEG. Some studies have suggested that patients with osteoarthritis and significant morning stiffness may have nocturnal myoclonus as well as alpha intrusion.

Chronic renal failure is associated with poor sleep at night, prolonged awakenings, and EDS. Improvements in sleep with decreased awakenings and an increase in Stage 3 and Stage 4 sleep are noted following dialysis.

Patients with *anorexia nervosa* often have sleep onset and sleep maintenance insomnia. They also are troubled with early morning awakenings. Sleep tends to improve as these patients gain weight.

Gastric acid secretion during sleep is increased up to 20 times greater than normal in patients with peptic ulcer disease. Nocturnal pain from peptic ulcer disease, as well as nocturnal gastroesophageal reflux or regurgitation, can disrupt sleep.

Chronic headache patients complain of insomnia and show a decrease in total sleep time along with frequent arousals. Patients with cluster or migraine headaches, or chronic paroxysmal hemicrania, frequently report that their headaches begin during sleep. Polysomnographic studies show that such headaches often start during, or shortly after, an episode of REM sleep.

Studies on asymptomatic HIV-positive patients have demonstrated an increase in slow wave sleep, especially in the second part of the night, as well as a decrease in sleep efficiency. Patients with *AIDS-related complex* and *symptomatic AIDS* may have complaints of both EDS and insomnia.

Many *toxic states* induced by medications or chemical exposure are associated with decreased and fragmented sleep. Carbon monoxide, mercury, arsenic, and cytotoxic chemotherapeutic agents for malignancies are a few of the compounds in this category.

Sleep disturbances can be seen as a *side effect* of a substantial number of commonly used pharmacological agents (see Table 6-1). The sleep complaint begins shortly after the onset of drug use, or following a dose increase, and decreases if the medication is withdrawn. Caffeine and nicotine may also disturb sleep in such a manner.

TABLE 6-1. **Common drugs with insomnia as a side effect**

Beta blockers	Stimulating tricyclics
Corticosteroids	Stimulants
ACTH	Thyroid hormones
MAO inhibitors	Oral contraceptives
Diphenylhydantoin	Antimetabolites
Calcium blockers	Some decongestants
α-Methyldopa	Thiazides
Bronchodilators	

Studies on patients who have undergone *surgical procedures*, or who are in *intensive care units*, demonstrate that these patients' sleep is fragmented, with frequent arousals, and contains very little Stage 3, Stage 4, or REM sleep. Many awakenings are due to nursing activities such as taking vital signs or administering medication. Nurses often overestimate the amount of sleep patients actually get.

TREATMENT OF SLEEP COMPLAINTS IN PATIENTS WITH MEDICAL ILLNESSES

The proper treatment in any patient with disordered sleep begins with the correct diagnosis. It is important to consider the effect of the primary medical illness on sleep, the consequences of therapies for the medical problem, and the possibility that coexistent primary sleep disorders exist.

If the sleep complaint is felt to be directly related to an underlying medical problem, the initial effort should be to improve that primary condition, as well as those symptoms disruptive to sleep. If the sleep complaint persists or worsens after controlling the medical problem, one must determine if aspects of the treatment modalities themselves may be contributing to the problem.

If the sleep complaint persists after resolution of the medical illness, it is likely that a primary sleep disorder may also exist.

Persistent psychophysiological insomnia commonly arises as a result of an acute medical illness. The presence of unsuspected primary sleep disorders such as nocturnal myoclonus or sleep apnea must also be considered. In some patients a polysomnographic evaluation is necessary to obtain a correct diagnosis.

Patients who are thought to have fibrositis often respond to small doses of amitriptyline (10–50 mg daily) or cyclobenzaprine (10 mg tid). Nonsteroidal anti-inflammatory agents sometimes are also of benefit. A PSG in these patients may be very useful in evaluating possible coexistent periodic limb movements of sleep (PLMS; nocturnal myoclonus). If PLMS is found, consideration should be given to use of a benzodiazepine hypnotic such as temazepam or clonazepam, and avoidance of tricyclic antidepressants.

Those patients who have insomnia associated with an acute medical illness and no other contraindication may be treated for a short time with hypnotics. Ideally, medications with a short half-life, such as triazolam 0.125 to 0.25 mg prior to bed, should be used.

The summary guidelines provided in Figure 6-2 may be helpful for treatment of insomnia in patients with medical illness.

■ PSYCHIATRIC DISORDERS AND SLEEP

Many psychiatric disorders are associated with prominent disturbances of sleep, most often in the form of insomnia, but occasionally in the form of excessive sleepiness, nightmares, or parasomnia-type behaviors. In this section we address the most frequently encountered sleep complaints found in the major groups of psychiatric disorders. The area of sleep disorders associated with substance abuse is considered separately in Chapter 3.

The complaint of insomnia is almost universally accompanied by some indication of psychological stress. MMPI evaluation of large groups of chronic insomniac patients has shown that as many as 75% of insomniac patients may be suffering from some degree of depression or dysthymia, and it has been estimated that 35–50% of chronic insomnia may be causally related to psychiatric illness. It is often not clear which comes first, the insomnia or the depression and/or anxiety. Patients often state, "You'd feel

> Step 1. Make a diagnosis.
>
> Step 2. Treat the medical illness first.
>
> Step 3. Consider if medications or treatment modalities contribute to the sleep complaint. If so, can the type of medication or dosing schedule be altered?
>
> Step 4. Consider the possibility of a primary sleep disorder. Formal PSG may be necessary.
>
> Step 5. In hospitalized patients the sleep needs should be considered when ordering vital sign checks, etc. Awakenings should be kept to a minimum.
>
> Step 6. Review principles of good sleep hygiene (see Chapter 3) with all patients.
>
> Step 7. Patients with acute medical illnesses and insomnia may be treated with hypnotics if no contraindications exist.

FIGURE 6-2. **Guidelines for treatment of insomnia in patients with medical illness.**

miserable and depressed too if you slept no more than I do." Similarly, it is not always clear whether anxiety precipitates insomnia, or whether a period of insomnia leads to anxiety about going to bed, only to lie awake and be unable to sleep. Such concerns underscore the importance of a thorough psychiatric evaluation as an essential part of a sleep history.

PSYCHIATRIC ASSESSMENT

Many of the important psychological variables can be picked up subtly during the interview by asking open-ended questions in such areas as what stressful events may be currently ongoing in the patient's life, or may have occurred around the time of initial difficulty with insomnia. One should also evaluate premorbid psychological and physical functioning. It is important to ask questions regarding childhood sleeping patterns, which can also elicit information about possible early developmental conflicts. Many patients fear being labeled a psychiatric patient. They may have biases that lead them to believe that if their sleep complaint is caused by something "that is all in your head," it is not truly a valid complaint. These patients may consequently steer away from talking about their depression or anxiety-related symptoms.

First create avenues for patients to openly express their concerns, and then directly ask difficult questions. Have suicidal ideas crossed your mind while lying awake? Have hopelessness and despondency set in around the fears of being unable to control insomnia? Have you had episodes of anxiety with physical symptoms such as tachycardia or hyperventilation? For many patients, the direct questions regarding symptoms of depression or panic disorder may relieve their fear of bringing up symptoms that they feel the physician may not want to hear, or are "too crazy to talk about."

An additional complication in obtaining the psychiatric history can be that many insomniac patients suffer from difficulties adequately expressing or even identifying their emotions, and thus find it hard to express feelings of anger or feelings about interpersonal conflicts.

It is frequently advisable to refrain from making final diagnostic conclusions on the basis of information obtained at the first visit. We find that many times patients are indeed right that their mood disorder symptoms or anxiety is secondary to their insomnia and that these symptoms may resolve with treatment of the sleep complaint. If one finds that psychiatric symptoms persist after appropriate behavioral and pharmacological intervention, one may consider that the psychiatric symptoms are likely to be primary and need their own specific treatment plan.

PSYCHIATRIC DISORDERS ASSOCIATED PRIMARILY WITH INSOMNIA

The following psychiatric disorders (Table 6-2) are those most frequently associated with insomnia.

SCHIZOPHRENIA

Deterioration of sleep, including a marked increase in frequency of nightmares, is common in schizophrenic patients before a psychotic break. Sleep EEGs have shown a tendency toward sleep fragmentation and a decrease in slow wave sleep in most schizo-

TABLE 6-2. **Psychiatric disorders frequently associated with sleep complaints**

Psychiatric disorders associated with insomnia

Schizophrenia

Major depression

Bipolar depression

Subaffective disorders

    Dysthymic disorder
    Hypomania
    Cyclothymic disorder
    Masked depression

Personality disorders

Anxiety-related disorders (see Table 6–3)

    Generalized anxiety disorder
    Panic disorder

Other disorders

    Somatoform disorders
    Posttraumatic stress disorder

Psychiatric disorders associated with EDS

Seasonal affective disorders

Atypical depression

phrenic patients. Acute schizophrenia has also been associated with shortened REM latency (4). In general, however, no diagnostically specific EEG sleep abnormalities are found in schizophrenia.

Preferred treatment of schizophrenia-related insomnia is use of a neuroleptic that will stabilize the psychotic symptoms and offer enough sedation to provide adequate sleep. It is best to avoid having to add benzodiazepines to the neuroleptic for long-term usage. It is important to make note of sleep problems that may develop later on in the lives of schizophrenic patients. If sleep later worsens, it is important to determine whether this deterioration is a side effect of medication, or is due to the onset of depression or the emergence of a syndrome such as sleep apnea. Chronic schizophrenic patients on long-term medication may gain an excessive amount of weight as a result of appetite stimulation, and can develop obstructive sleep apnea secondary to this weight gain. In these cases intervention such as weight loss, nasal continuous positive airway pressure, or addition of a tricyclic may be required.

MAJOR DEPRESSION

Greater than 10% of our population will suffer an episode of major depression during their adult life, and 90–95% of these people will suffer extremely disordered sleep during this bout of depression. Insomnia is the most frequent complaint. Early morning awakening with difficulty returning to sleep is common in, but not pathognomonic of, depression.

The insomnia of major depression has a very high likelihood of response to tricyclic antidepressants, so it is vital to never miss the diagnosis. A useful mnemonic is DSIGECAPS, which would be a reminder that the prescription for *D*epression would be written *sig*: *ECAPS*, standing for the following:

*D*epressed mood
*S*leeplessness
*I*nterests—decreased
*G*uilt
*E*nergy—decreased
*C*oncentration—decreased

*A*ppetite—diminished
*P*sychomotor agitation or retardation
*S*uicidal ideation

The presence of five of these nine symptoms for 2 weeks or more, including the presence of either depressed mood or loss of interest, fulfills the criteria for the diagnosis of major depression.

Nocturnal polysomnographic studies of depressed patients show a tendency toward a decreasing continuity of sleep and decreases in delta sleep, as well as a characteristic decrease in nocturnal REM latency (time between sleep onset and the onset of the first REM period). There may be an increase in phasic activity (e.g., REM density) and, often, in duration of the first REM period (5). Thus in major depression REM sleep occurs earlier and is more intense, more like the REM sleep seen in the early morning hours of nondepressed individuals. These findings have suggested that the REM sleep rhythm may be phase-advanced in major depression.

The sleep EEG has been helpful in predicting response to medication. Patients with major depression or subaffective disorders who have shortened REM latency, which increases in length with the administration of tricyclic antidepressants, are more likely to be positive responders to tricyclic antidepressants (6).

Sedative tricyclics may be especially helpful in depressed patients with insomnia. Nortriptyline is often a good initial candidate because of its moderate side effect profile and low likelihood of causing daytime sedation. Occasionally, the less-sedating tricyclics may aggravate insomnia, and therefore a shift to a more sedating tricyclic would be in order. It must be remembered that tricyclics can cause or aggravate PLMS or nocturnal myoclonus (see Chapter 3). Switching to a more purely serotonin-potentiating antidepressant (e.g., doxepin or trazodone) may be helpful in those patients whose PLMS are aggravated or have become symptomatic.

Because of the several-week lag period between the beginning of drug administration and therapeutic response, there may be a need for the temporary use of a benzodiazepine for sleep. After an early stabilization period it is best to try to avoid the long-term use of benzodiazepines. Most patients will obtain adequate sleep with the antidepressant alone. It may be difficult to convince patients who have had very severe or chronic episodes of depression to reduce or stop a hypnotic medication. If the side effects are not severe it is often best to avoid tapering or cessation of the medication until the patient feels comfortable with the change.

Sleep deprivation has been found to improve mood in as many as 50% of depressive patients. One theory is that the insomnia symptom is the body's attempt to normalize mood. This may account for the observation that taking a hypnotic to improve the insomnia may occasionally aggravate the depression. Many affective disorders are associated with early morning awakening, and the loss of early morning sleep selectively reduces REM sleep, which appears to be elevated in many depressions. Again, this may be evidence of an internal homeostatic mechanism at work.

Psychotherapy for the depressed patient is helpful, and should be supportive and provide help to work through loss or bereavement issues, to identify and explain maladaptive patterns, to help boost self-esteem, to help the patient to appropriately express anger, and to decrease the tendency toward self-criticism.

BIPOLAR DISORDER

In the acute manic phase, bipolar patients will have sharply reduced sleep times, but they will have a great deal of energy despite the minimal amount of sleep. Recent sleep studies suggest that sleep during the manic phase may exhibit REM changes similar to those seen in depression (7). During the depressed phases these same patients may suffer from hypersomnia with excessive sleep but complain still of fatigue and lethargy. Appropriate regulation of sleep in the bipolar patient is important because sleep deprivation can be a trigger for manic episodes (8). During the acute phase the use of benzodiazepines or neuroleptics with sedative properties is usually the most effective treatment of the sleep problem until the patient can be stabilized on an antimanic drug such as lithium.

OTHER MOOD-RELATED DISORDERS

This is a heterogeneous and poorly defined group, sometimes

termed "subaffective disorders," which includes dysthymic disorder, hypomania, cyclothymia, masked depression, and certain personality disorders. These disorders are grouped together both because they do not fit into any other clear-cut diagnostic categories, and because they frequently include the presence of an affective component that may respond to antidepressants even though the patient may not fit the formal criteria for major depression.

Dysthymic disorder is diagnosed by the presence of at least 2 years of depressed mood accompanied by symptoms such as abnormal sleep, appetite, decreased energy, decreased self-esteem, hopelessness, or poor concentration. A significant number of dysthymic patients have shortened REM latencies (9). This group of patients seem to have a particularly good response to tricyclic antidepressants. Nonresponders may benefit from supportive psychotherapy and help in increasing socialization and the ability to express emotion.

Hypomania and cyclothymia are both syndromes in which there may be evidence of decreased sleep, but the patients will not necessarily complain of the insomnia because of increased energy. The cyclothymic patient may only complain of the insomnia during the dysthymic phase. It is important to differentiate these syndromes from disorders resulting from substance abuse or withdrawal (see Chapter 3). Treatment may include lithium for the hyperactivity, or carbamazepine (Tegretol) for the hyperactivity and explosive behavior. Cyclic antidepressants may be useful, especially in those patients with childhood histories of hyperactivity.

Masked depression may not be a distinct category, but there is some suggestion that a relationship may exist between insomnia and subclinical depressions (10).

PERSONALITY DISORDERS

Borderline personality disorder patients studied with polysomnography have frequently been found to have decreased REM latency (11, 12). Patients with shortened REM latencies were more likely to respond to tricyclic antidepressants, with benefits in both mood and sleep, than were the patients with normal REM latencies.

ANXIETY-RELATED DISORDERS

Table 6-3 displays one way to conceptualize a continuum of anxiety-related syndromes as they relate to sleep complaints and their treatment. The disorders listed range from least severe (psychophysiological insomnia) to most severe (panic disorder). We do not mean to imply that there is a continuity or singularity of mechanism underlying these disorders, but rather that all have an element of anxiety in their presentation and all may adversely influence sleep. We present them as a continuum because the symptoms often tend to be overall fairly similar in type, if not severity (e.g., fear, being easily panicked, tendency to feel fatigued or depleted, hypervigilance, and a tendency toward rumination).

Anxiety-related disorders are frequently associated with a number of physical complaints, including autonomic hyperactivity, gastrointestinal distress, weakness, light-headedness, paresthesias, and headaches. The most severe anxiety-related disorders, panic disorder and obsessive-compulsive disorder, will usually need medication in addition to other behavioral and psychotherapeutic interventions. The continuum of listed disorders requires individual tailoring of the regimen to that which the patient responds to and feels most comfortable with. Table 6-3 also includes a hierarchy of treatments generally used with these disorders. There is a preference to try to allow treatment to occur without medication and with the least expense to the patient whenever possible.

Panic disorder, the most severe anxiety-related disorder, is characterized by discrete spontaneous episodes of intense fear or panic that are often accompanied by symptoms of autonomic hyperarousal such as tachycardia, shortness of breath, sweating, nausea, and increased muscle tension. The attacks may last only a few minutes, but they can have a devastating effect on the sufferer both from the immediate disruption and from the sustained fear of recurrence.

Panic attacks occur most often during the day but may occur at night. Nocturnal attacks will often wake the patient from sleep with symptoms of tachycardia and shortness of breath, which may be mistaken as symptoms of a sleep apnea syndrome. There are no sleep laboratory findings specific for panic disorder, unless

TABLE 6-3. **Continuum of anxiety-related disorders with frequent insomnia complaint**

Disorder	Comments	Treatment
1. Psychophysiological insomnia	Negative conditioning to own bedroom; sleeps better away from home.	Sleep restriction; behavioral techniques; perhaps medication (see Chapter 3).
2. Sleep phobia	Negative conditioning to any sleep.	Sleep restriction and prn benzodiazepine.
3. Nocturnal separation anxiety	Fears loss of connectedness with world.	Rigid A.M. arising time; insight-oriented psychotherapy; consider low-dose tricyclic.
4. Nocturnal fear of loss of control	Daytime obsessive-compulsive traits; ineffective ability to control sleep.	May need tricyclic or prn benzodiazepine to regain control; supportive psychotherapy.
5. Generalized anxiety disorder	Chronic worrier, persistent hyperarousal.	Milder cases respond to behavioral techniques; more severe cases may need benzodiazepines or tricyclics.
6. Obsessive-compulsive disorder	Lifestyle of developed behaviors to control anxieties.	MAO inhibitors, tricyclics; consider psychotherapy or behavioral therapy techniques.
7. Panic disorder symptoms	e.g., Tachycardia and/or shortness of breath plus insomnia.	May respond best to benzodiazepines such as alprazolam, as antidepressants increase heart rate and may aggravate condition early on.
8. Panic disorder	Paroxysms of anxiety and fear, with autonomic hyperarousal.	MAO inhibitors, cyclic antidepressants, benzodiazepines; behavioral therapy; psychotherapy.

a full-blown attack is recorded complete with tachycardia, increased respiration, and panic.

The use of a moderately sedating tricyclic antidepressant at a once-daily dosage may benefit sleep as a result of the agent's sedative effect, as well as control the panic episodes throughout the day. Monoamine oxidase inhibitors (MAOIs) are of significant value to some patients. Dosages of MAOIs should be given early in the day to try to minimize sleep disruption. The panic disorder patient with a primary complaint of insomnia may, however, be an inappropriate candidate for an MAOI. Many panic disorder sufferers are very sensitive to medication side effects and seem to do better on benzodiazepines such as alprazolam or clonazepam.

SUBPANIC ANXIETY OR PANIC DISORDER SYMPTOM ATTACKS

Certain patients who do not qualify for the formal diagnosis of panic disorder will have subclinical symptom attacks, which may include shortness of breath or tachycardia, that appear to lead to a secondary insomnia. Many times these patients will complain of little or no anxiety throughout the day but feel that these episodes happen more commonly in the evening and significantly aggravate sleep. Beta blockers may limit tachycardiac symptoms but offer no benefit for the insomnia or the overall syndrome. Low-dose benzodiazepines such as alprazolam or clonazepam can often be given in a once-daily dosage in the evening as an effective means of controlling both the physical symptoms and the insomnia, even with persistent usage.

SOMATOFORM DISORDER

The patient who somatizes appears to convert an emotional problem into a physical complaint. Insomnia as a somatized complaint is probably second in frequency only to headaches. The typical patient with somatoform disorder will actually have a broad array of physical complaints, which over time become quite fixed, and for which no underlying medical illness, positive laboratory tests, or adequate treatment can apparently be found. These patients are very poor at expressing their emotions and may suffer from alexithymia or absence of words for emotions.

Many of these patients have grown up in an environment of

physical or emotional abuse or neglect, and symptoms may be the patient's perceived link to a source of caring or concern. They may become angry if the physician tries to reassure them that they are going to be alright. Attempts to minimize the seriousness of their illness may only increase the tenacity with which these patients will cling to the symptoms. It is very important, with a patient who somatizes, to not prescribe sleeping medications without a very clear understanding as to when, and for how long, the medication will be prescribed. If the physician feels the medication is not likely to solve the problem, it would be best not to start medication in the first place. It is best to indicate to the patient that you recognize his or her frustration with the illness, and that you respect the treatments he or she has previously received and will not make rapid changes in any current medication regimens. The patient should be scheduled for regular follow-up appointments. This follow-up period will meet some of the patient's dependency needs, through a continued attachment with the physician, such that the patient may be able to reduce reliance on the physical complaint to meet his or her needs. Inpatient hospitalization may at times be the treatment of choice for the somatizing insomniac patient who is unresponsive to all other treatments (13).

POSTTRAUMATIC STRESS DISORDER

Posttraumatic stress disorder (PTSD) is a syndrome of anxiety and chronic hyperarousal related to preoccupation with and reexperiencing of severely traumatic or life-threatening events such as war experiences, serious accidents, and physical or sexual assaults. It is often characterized by repetitive traumatic memories of the original event, preoccupation with the original trauma, and frequent reexposure to the traumatic event through flashbacks, nightmares, and night terrors. Chronic insomnia secondary to the hyperarousal is very common. The PTSD patient may become socially isolated and at times may resort to the use of drugs or alcohol to suppress the traumatic memories and tormented wakefulness.

The nocturnal PSG of the PTSD patient is characterized by shortened sleep time, frequent awakenings, and frequent night terror-type arousals from slow wave sleep. Most of the night terror-type events occur during the first third of the night, and they are often accompanied by verbalization, emotion, and more dream-like content than is usually seen in night terrors. Nightmares are associated with REM sleep and generally occur later in the night.

Most PTSD patients can benefit from some form of psychotherapy, either individual or group, especially early in the course of the syndrome. The ability to talk about their traumatic experience seems to be quite helpful, and may, over time, diminish the continued anxiety and hyperarousal. Early in treatment, for very severe cases, it is usually necessary to use medication to suppress night terror activity, suppress REM nightmares, and help provide relief with the chronic insomnia. Tricyclic antidepressants, at an antidepressant dose, are often the preferred mode of treatment. Other medications that have shown occasional usefulness in PTSD include MAOIs, carbamazepine, lithium, and propranolol. Benzodiazepines may be helpful, but because of the chronicity of the disorder, tolerance may develop.

PSYCHIATRIC DISORDERS ASSOCIATED WITH EXCESSIVE DAYTIME SLEEPINESS

SEASONAL AFFECTIVE DISORDERS

Seasonal affective disorders (SADs) are disorders of mood, presenting as either depression, hypomania, or mania, that are very closely linked with certain seasons. SADs may be related to a circadian rhythm disturbance precipitated by the changes in the length of the day. A typical case might be a female in her 30s who begins to show evidence of depression and excessive sleepiness in October and November (in the Northern Hemisphere), as the days begin getting shorter. The depression might last throughout the winter, and only begin improving as the days become longer in the spring. Some patients will report the opposite symptoms in the spring and summer, with the development of hypomanic symptoms, including irritability, decreased sleep, and hyperactivity. The majority of the depressive symptoms tend to be atypical in nature, with increased sleep time, decreased energy, increased appetite, a carbohydrate craving, weight increase, decreased activity, and daytime drowsiness. The diagnosis is made in those patients who have had a history of at least one major depressive episode and who show at least two occurrences of fall/winter depression with nondepressed periods during the spring and summer. In addition to this typical SAD, there appears to be a reverse SAD that consists of a hypomanic period during the winter, with the period of depression occurring during the spring and summer. Patients with spring/summer depression appear, however, to report decreased sleep and decreased appetite. There are apparently no clear PSG findings to distinguish SAD.

SADs have been found to respond to 2 hours of bright-light (2,500 lux) exposure immediately upon awakening in the morning. Commercial light units are available to provide this intensity light. The unit is normally placed about 3 feet from the patient, who is instructed to look up at the light once per minute. Response should occur within a matter of days and should be complete within 2 weeks. If the patient does not respond to treatment, increases in light exposure or shifting light exposure to evening hours should be considered. SAD patients who are suffering from early morning awakening should begin their trial of light exposure in the evening. Psychotropic drugs such as tricyclic antidepressants, MAOIs, and lithium may be useful treatment adjuncts (14).

ATYPICAL DEPRESSION

Atypical depression differs from the usual presentation of major depression in that patients tend to exhibit excessive sleepiness, lethargy, increased appetite, carbohydrate craving, and inability to initiate enjoyable activities, but often an ability to enjoy activities initiated by others. Symptoms in common with major depression include poor concentration, decrease in energy, low self-esteem, and suicidal ideation.

Atypical depression may be responsive to MAOIs such as phenelzine. MAOIs tend to be somewhat activating, and may reduce sleep time, which can be of benefit for those patients who present with excessive sleep as a complaint (15).

It should be remembered that major depression can also present with hypersomnolence, and that defense mechanisms found in many psychiatric disorders can include hypersomnolence and drowsiness as a form of psychological withdrawal. There is evidence that depression in adolescence more commonly presents as EDS and hypersomnolence (16).

■ REFERENCES

1. Williams RL: Sleep disturbances in various medical and surgical conditions, in Sleep Disorders: Diagnosis and Treatment. Edited by Williams RL, Karacan I. New York, John Wiley, 1978, pp 285–301
2. Dunleavy D, Oswald I, Brown P, et al: Hyperthyroidism, sleep and growth hormone. Electroencephalogr Clin Neurophysiol 36:159–263, 1974
3. Moldofsky H: Sleep and fibrositis syndrome. Rheum Dis Clin North Am 15:91–103, 1989
4. Zarcone VP, Benson KL, Berger PA: Abnormal rapid eye movement latencies in schizophrenia. Arch Gen Psychiatry 44:455–458, 1981
5. Cable P, Foster FG, Kupfer DJ: Electroencephalographic sleep diagnosis of primary depression. Arch Gen Psychiatry 33:1124–1127, 1976
6. Kupfer DJ, Spiker DG, Rossi A, et al: Recent diagnostic and treatment advances in REM sleep depression, in Treatment of Depression: Old Controversies and New Approaches. Edited by Clayton P, Barrett J. New York, Raven Press, 1983
7. Post RM, Stoddard FJ, Gillin FC, et al: Slow and rapid laterationi in motor activity, sleep and biochemistry in a cycling manic-depressive patient. Arch Gen Psychiatry 34:470–477, 1976
8. Wehr TA, Sack DA, Rosenthal NE: Sleep reduction as a final common pathway in the genesis of mania. Am J Psychiatry 144:201–204, 1987
9. Akiskal H, Lemmi H, Dickson H, et al: Chronic depressions: II. Sleep EEG differentiation of primary dysthymic disorder from anxious depression. J Affective Disord 6:287–295, 1984
10. Gillin JC: The sleep therapies of depression. Prog Neuropsychopharmacol Biol Psychiatry 7:351–364, 1983
11. McNamara E, Reynolds CF, Soloff PH, et al: EEG sleep evaluation of depression in borderline patients. Am J Psychiatry 141:182–186, 1984
12. Reynolds CF, Soloff PH, Kupfer DJ, et al: Depression in borderline patients: a prospective EEG study. Psychiatry Res 14:1–15, 1985
13. Tan TL, Kales JD, Kales A, et al: Inpatient multidimensional management of treatment resistent insomnia. Psychosomatics 28: 266–272, 1987
14. Rosenthal NE, Wehr TA: Seasonal affective disorders. Psychiatr Ann 17:670–674, 1987

15. Quitkin FM, Schwartz D, Liebowitz MR, et al: Atypical depressives: a preliminary report of antidepressant response and sleep patterns. Psychopharmacol Bull 18:78–80, 1982
16. Hawkins D, Tub J, Vande Castle R: Extended sleep (hypersomnia) in young depressives. Am J Psychiatry 142:405–410, 1985

■ ADDITIONAL READING

Dicicco B, Cooper J, Waldhorn R: Sleep disorders in medical illness. Psychiatr Med 4:113–147, 1987

7 USE OF SEDATIVE-HYPNOTIC AGENTS

Sedative-hypnotic agents designed for the treatment of insomnia remain among the most widely prescribed medications. In the past they have too frequently been misused, and abused, based upon both a lack of understanding of drug effects on sleep, and the fact that very different sleep disorders, requiring different treatments, may present with similar symptoms. This situation is fortunately changing as we learn more about sleep disorders medicine and about the effects of drugs on sleep.

It is a truism that drugs which affect sleep also change sleep. This fact can be useful in, for example, the use of benzodiazepines to suppress Stage 3 and Stage 4 sleep and associated parasomnias, or the use of REM-suppressant drugs to treat certain REM-related disorders. The substantial REM suppression encountered with the barbiturates, however, frequently leads to difficulties in withdrawing these agents, because of the associated REM rebound accompanied by frightening nightmares.

The most appropriate use of sedative-hypnotic agents is for the treatment of transient insomnia, such as stress-, altitude-, or jet lag-related insomnia (as described in Chapter 3), or for short-term treatment of other symptomatic insomnias, such as those accompanying medical disorders. Patient education is a most important component of any hypnotic therapeutic regimen. Patients should be informed about the effects of drugs on sleep, the possible development of tolerance, and the risks of drug dependency. It should be emphasized to the patient that the goal of hypnotic use is to increase alertness and energy in the daytime, and that the ability for a hypnotic to help in this respect is probably limited to several weeks of continual usage. If it is expected at the outset that a longer period of treatment will be necessary, it is preferable to plan intermittent use of two to four doses per week. In this way the patient can be assured of at least several good nights of sleep each week, which in turn will lower anxiety, while the risk of developing tolerance will be diminished. As a general rule it is recommended that no more than 20 doses of medication be prescribed during any one month if possible, and that the lowest effective dose be prescribed. The patient should be reminded that elevating dosages above the typical therapeutic level seldom results in sustained improvement in sleep or daytime functioning. Patients using hypnotics should remain in contact with their physician, who should maintain an active role in medication control.

We should keep in mind that a large number of chronic insomnias are the result of a transient insomnia for which the patient makes an inappropriate behavioral adaptation that prevents the insomnia from resolving. One common behavioral maladaptation is the persistent use of sedative-hypnotic agents (which may be iatrogenic) or alcohol (which has been estimated to be the major cause of greater than 10% of chronic insomnias). On the other hand, failure to provide appropriate symptomatic treatment of short-term insomnia can also lead to a more chronic insomnia.

■ CHOICE OF A HYPNOTIC AGENT

Primary pharmacological factors to be considered with respect to hypnotic agents include (a) therapeutic index (safety), (b) rate of absorption, (c) rate of metabolism (half-life), and (d) presence of possible drug interactions.

BENZODIAZEPINE HYPNOTIC AGENTS

Benzodiazepines are the agent of choice for short-term treatment of insomnia. Their major advantages include greater safety because of the relatively favorable therapeutic index (margin between therapeutic and lethal dosages), prolonged effectiveness, and less inducement of hepatic microsomal enzymes.

Benzodiazepines as a group are probably effective as hypnotics for a number of weeks of continual usage (although intermittent use is preferred). These agents tend to suppress Stage 3 and Stage 4 sleep, which leads to their occasional use in the treatment of Stage 3- and Stage 4-related parasomnias. They slightly diminish REM sleep, but not to the same extent as do barbiturates. The three benzodiazepine agents currently approved for hypnotic use are listed in Table 7-1. Substantial differences in half-life, with triazolam having a short half-life, temazepam an intermediate one, and flurazepam a long one, make these three hypnotic agents useful in different clinical situations (1).

TRIAZOLAM

Triazolam is the drug of choice for sleep onset insomnia because of its relatively rapid mode of action and rapid elimination. Triazolam may be administered sublingually, with an almost immediate onset of action. It may also be taken relatively late at night (e.g., midnight or 1:00 A.M.), after the patient realizes he or

TABLE 7-1. **Currently approved benzodiazepine hypnotics**

Drug	Usual dosage (mg)	Half-life of active metabolites (hours)	Duration of sedative effect (hours)
Triazolam (Halcion)	0.125–0.25	2–3	4–6
Temazepam (Restoril)	15–30	8–10	6–8
Flurazepam (Dalmane)	15–30	50–200	12 or more

she is unable to get to sleep, and still permit 5–6 hours of sleep without morning hangover. Because most of the drug is gone by morning, and virtually all of it has disappeared by afternoon, this drug will not accumulate in the body and offers optimal daytime alertness. This characteristic can be especially valuable in the elderly, who may have decreased metabolism, or competition for metabolism from other medications. Major drawbacks of a quickly eliminated drug such as triazolam are relatively shorter hypnotic effect, occasional early morning insomnia (due to an intranight rebound), and occasionally a morning withdrawal effect that can result in agitation or aggravation of daytime anxiety (2). After continuous use of the drug for several weeks, sudden discontinuation may result in a rebound insomnia lasting several days. A dose of 0.125 mg is recommended, although 0.25 mg may be required. Doses of 0.5 mg or more may be associated with anterograde amnesia and are not recommended.

TEMAZEPAM

Temazepam is an appropriate hypnotic for those patients with nocturnal awakenings. Some patients may experience a bit of morning grogginess, but few patients will experience a significant buildup of blood level over time. A drawback of temazepam is its relatively slow onset of action, due to slow absorption, which can at times be 1–2 hours. This characteristic necessitates administration up to an hour before bedtime. Complaints of rebound insomnia will likely occur at termination of regular nightly usage, but this insomnia will possibly be delayed for a night or two. A dose of 15 mg should be tried first; 30 mg may be necessary in some cases.

FLURAZEPAM

Flurazepam has a slowly eliminated metabolite, desalkylflurazepam, with a half-life ranging from 40 to 100 hours or more, which accounts for the tendency for buildup with regular administration. This agent is of greatest value for patients suffering from significant daytime anxiety as well as insomnia. Its advantages are that it provides a particularly long sleep period and has been demonstrated to be effective for at least several weeks of nightly use. Flurazepam can curb daytime anxiety, and at the time of discontinuance there is minimal initial rebound insomnia. A later rebound insomnia, accompanied by increased anxiety, may be noted several weeks following discontinuation when long-half-life metabolites are eliminated. The disadvantages of the long elimination half-life of the drug are diminution of daytime alertness and potentially toxic blood levels with prolonged administration. In many cases the daytime sedation can defeat the advantage of improved nocturnal sleep; this can be potentially serious in those individuals with daytime jobs requiring high degrees of alertness. Flurazepam should be used with caution in the elderly, in whom persistent use has been associated with daytime sedation, and motor and cognitive impairment (3).

OTHER BENZODIAZEPINE AGENTS

The sedative or hypnotic use of those benzodiazepines that are usually prescribed as anxiolytics is certainly appropriate, and at times desired. Table 7-2 provides information on anxiolytic benzodiazepine drugs that also have hypnotic effects. For the patient with chronic anxiety who may need a benzodiazepine for symptom relief, it is not necessary to prescribe a second medication for sleep. It is preferable to adjust the daytime dosage so that a significant amount of anxiolytic is given at bedtime to promote adequate sleep.

INTERACTION WITH OTHER DRUGS

Benzodiazepines as a group do not appear to enhance or impair the metabolism of other drugs. However, the CNS-depressant effects of alcohol are additive with benzodiazepines, and patients should be cautioned about possible additive effects. Ethanol can slow the hepatic metabolism of benzodiazepines, thus enhancing or prolonging their effect. This is of special concern with the longer-half-life agents and in the elderly or in those with compromised liver function. Cimetidine also impairs the metabolism of most benzodiazepines, except for those metabolized exclusively by conjugation.

NONBENZODIAZEPINE HYPNOTIC AGENTS

There are several additional drugs or groups of drugs that have occasional usefulness as hypnotics.

TABLE 7-2. **Other benzodiazepines frequently used for their sedative-hypnotic effects**

Drug	Typical bedtime dosage range (mg)	Elimination half-life of drug and active metabolites (hours)
Chlordiazepoxide (Librium)	5–25	5–30
Lorazepam (Ativan)	0.5–3	10–20
Clonazepam (Clonopin)	0.5–4	20–40
Diazepam (Valium)	2–10	20–100
Clorazepate (Tranxene)	7.5–15	30–200
Alprazolam (Xanax)	0.25–2	12–20
Oxazepam (Serax)	10–25	5–15

CHLORAL HYDRATE

Chloral hydrate was historically one of the first hypnotics available, and still can have some usefulness at 0.5 to 1 g. With proper dosage adjustment, it is rare for habituation to develop, and chloral hydrate generally does not cause adverse effects on sleep architecture. Major drawbacks include a tendency for gastric irritation and skin rash, and a tendency to interfere with concomitant usage of drugs such as phenytoin and warfarin or coumadin. A further drawback involves the induction of hepatic microsomal enzymes. Some find it a very helpful hypnotic, while others have found that after 2 weeks' administration its effect is only slightly better than placebo.

BARBITURATE COMPOUNDS

A number of barbiturate compounds were the sedative-hypnotics of choice prior to benzodiazepines becoming available. Some physicians continue to use the barbiturate medications out of habit, but usage in general has dropped dramatically. Major drawbacks include relatively low therapeutic index; induction of hepatic microsomal enzyme systems, which alters (increases) the metabolic rate of other drugs; relatively short duration of effectiveness; significant distortion of sleep; and potentially dangerous withdrawal and side effects. Because of the relatively brief period of hypnotic effectiveness (a relatively few days), patients often escalate the dosage very rapidly. Attempts to discontinue the medication can initiate quite unpleasant withdrawal effects, such as frightening nightmares associated with REM rebound, which may cause the patient to continue the drug and possibly increase its dose. More serious withdrawal effects include seizures. Barbiturates are much more likely than the benzodiazepines to produce addiction, and they are much more lethal if used in suicide attempts by overdose.

MORE RARELY USED NONBARBITURIC AGENTS

Several nonbarbituric agents have also historically been used as hypnotics; but with the advent of benzodiazepines these agents are no longer felt to be appropriate choices as sedative-hypnotics, except perhaps in special and limited cases. These agents include ethchlorvynol (Placidyl), glutethimide (Doriden), methaqualone (Parest), and methyprylon (Noludar).

L-TRYPTOPHAN

A comment is in order concerning L-tryptophan, which, while not a hypnotic, may occasionally be useful for some patients with mild insomnia. A major appeal is that it is an essential amino acid and a precursor of serotonin, which is thought to be an important neurotransmitter for certain slow wave sleep systems. As the typical diet includes ½–2 grams of L-tryptophan, the use of 3–4 grams offers little significant deviation from the daily diet. The main advantage of L-tryptophan seems to be an occasional decrease in sleep latency rather than any prolongation of sleep time (4). There are high concentrations of L-tryptophan in milk and in chicken, both of which have been subjectively reported as facilitating nocturnal sleep (thus the late tryptophan snack as part of good sleep hygiene). L-Tryptophan is frequently the agent of choice in the treatment of insomnia in a substance-abusing population or among those seeking a more "natural" treatment.

While tryptophan has been claimed to be the "natural hypnotic," and is often recommended in the popular press for the treatment of a number of sleep-related disorders, including insomnia, in fact its effectiveness in chronic insomnia remains to be empirically demonstrated in well-controlled double-blind studies. Nonetheless, its occasional effectiveness in insomnia, and its demonstrated effectiveness in decreasing sleep latency under certain conditions in noninsomniac individuals, probably merit its trial in some chronic insomniac patients. The safety and efficacy of long-term use of high doses of tryptophan have yet to be demonstrated, however, and hepatic ultrastructural changes (of unclear significance) have been described in animals following high-dose administration of tryptophan (5).

ANTIHISTAMINES

Antihistamines such as diphenhydramine (25–50 mg) can often be of value as a sedative. Generally these agents are not preferred over benzodiazepines, for while they may decrease sleep latency, they have not been shown to increase total sleep time. The two major areas of usage would be in the substance-abusing population, in which case one should not take habituating substances, or in treatment of insomnia in the patient who is also suffering from allergy or itching.

TRICYCLICS

Occasionally a sedating tricyclic such as amitriptyline, doxepin, or nortriptyline used in the range of 10–100 mg is a useful sleep-inducing agent. Table 7-3 lists dosages and advantages of commonly used sedative antidepressants.

A major advantage of the tricyclics is the lack of development of tolerance over time. However, major drawbacks include anticholinergic side effects and aggravation of periodic limb movements of sleep (nocturnal myoclonus). Such medications are predominantly used in patients with previous depressive episodes, dysthymic-type disorders, or some anxiety disorders, and in patients with a history of hyperactivity as a child. Tricyclics are potent suppressors of REM sleep; this accounts for their occa-

TABLE 7-3. Currently available heterocyclic antidepressants

Drug	Trade name	Usual daily dose (mg)	Sedation	Advantages in sleep-disordered patient	Disadvantages in sleep-disordered patient
Amitriptyline	Elavil	150–300	+++	Increased sedation.	Increased anticholinergic, increased daytime sedation.
Nortriptyline	Pamelor Aventyl	75–125	++	Decreased daytime drowsiness, anticholinergic.	Not enough sedation.
Protriptyline	Vivactil	30–40	0	Activating for some narcoleptic patients.	Increased anticholinergic.
Imipramine	Tofranil	150–200	++	Decreased daytime sedation.	Orthostatic hypotension.
Desipramine	Norpramin Pertofrane	150–250	+	Minimal sedation for patients with narcolepsy or night terrors.	Can aggravate insomnia.
Trimipramine	Surmontil	150–200	+++	Increased sedation.	Over-sedation, increased anticholinergic.
Doxepin	Sinequan	150–250	+++	Increased sedation.	Increased anticholinergic.
Trazodone	Desyrel	150–400	+++	Increased sedation, decreased anticholinergic, decreased aggravation of myoclonus.	Increased orthostasis, nausea, and priapism.
Fluoxetine	Prozac	20–60	0	Decreased sedation, decreased anticholinergic, decreased appetite.	Can aggravate insomnia.

Note. 0, None; +, slight; ++, moderate; +++, high.

sional usefulness in the treatment of REM-related parasomnias and posttraumatic stress disorder.

■ LONGER-TERM USE OF SEDATIVE-HYPNOTIC AGENTS

While there clearly are appropriate times for long-term usage of sedative-hypnotics, these instances are relatively rare, and the large majority of persistent sedative-hypnotic use can be avoided by thorough sleep evaluations with more accurate diagnoses and by paying greater attention to behavioral techniques. For those patients who do in fact need prolonged treatment for sleep complaints, sedative-hypnotic agents are not necessarily the best choice.

Patients with chronic anxiety disorders with associated sleep complaints are perhaps best managed by administration of a sufficient anxiolytic agent, with appropriate hs dosages both to diminish daytime anxiety and to decrease nocturnal arousal sufficiently for sleep. In addition to responding to benzodiazepine anxiolytics, these patients also often respond to tricyclic antidepressants, to which they will develop little or no tolerance.

Some elderly patients may require relatively long-term hypnotic use. The elderly have a decreased ability to maintain continuity of sleep, frequent spontaneous arousals, and an increase in frequency of periodic limb movements and apneas. They, as well, often experience increased pain associated with chronic illness, take other medications, and have worries and anxieties that can lead to a multifactorial and difficult-to-treat insomnia complaint (see Chapter 8). While these patients are just as susceptible to the development of tolerance to sedative-hypnotics as any one else, they may be relieved at having the opportunity to use several doses of medication per week to guarantee predictable refreshing nights of sleep without substantial risk of development of tolerance. Short-half-life benzodiazepine hypnotics are preferred in this population.

Other chronic medical conditions may also require long-term hypnotic use. Each case must be evaluated individually, using the least medication possible and maximizing the use of behavioral techniques whenever possible.

REFERENCES

1. Greenblatt DJ, Divoll M, Abernathy DR, et al: Benzodiazepine hypnotics: kinetic and therapeutic options. Sleep 5:S18-S27, 1982
2. Kales A, Soldatos CR, Bixler EO, et al: Early morning insomnia with rapidly eliminated benzodiazepines. Science 220:95–97, 1983
3. Kramer M, Schoen LS: Problems in the use of long-acting hypnotics in older persons. J Clin Psychiatry 45:176–177, 1984
4. Hartmann E, Spinweaver CL: Sleep induced by L-tryptophan: effect of dosages within the normal dietary intake. J Nerv Ment Dis 167:497–499, 1979
5. Trulson ME, Sampson HW: Ultrastructural changes of the liver following L-tryptophan ingestion in rats. J Nutr 116:1109–1115, 1986

ADDITIONAL READINGS

Mendelson WB: The Use and Misuse of Sleeping Pills. New York, Plenum Press, 1980

National Institute of Mental Health, National Institutes of Health: Drugs and Insomnia. Consensus Development Conference Summary, Vol 4, No 10. Bethesda, MD, U.S. Department of Health and Human Services, 1984

8 SPECIAL PROBLEMS AND POPULATIONS

SLEEP PROBLEMS IN CHILDREN

This section addresses the most frequently encountered sleep problems in infants and children, and includes both symptomatic presentations, and sleep disturbances frequently accompanying specific diagnostic categories in infants and children. As with adult sleep disturbances, it is important to first carefully assess whether there might be some medical condition associated with a child's sleep complaint, and if so to treat this condition as appropriate.

INFANTS AND CHILDREN WHO DO NOT (OR CANNOT) SLEEP

Ferber (1) makes an important point about insomnia in infants and children:

> There is an important difference between the "insomnias" of the young child and that of the adult. An insomniac adult remains awake despite *his own* desires and efforts to fall asleep. A sleepless infant or toddler also remains awake, but in this case it is despite *his parents'* desires and efforts to have him fall asleep. "Insomnia" as experienced by adults probably does not occur before middle childhood. (p. 141)

The majority of sleep problems in infancy result from either parental difficulties in handling potentially time-limited sleep disturbances that then become chronic disturbances of sleep habits, or sleep disturbances found in somewhat atypical infants.

Most infants develop a 24-hour sleep-wake rhythm ("settle") by the age of 16 weeks (range 3–6 months), and are by then sleeping fairly well throughout the night and are awake predominantly during the daytime hours. It is difficult to be sure there is a sleep problem in an infant prior to 6 months because of normal variability in settling. Occasional nighttime awakenings are to be expected thereafter, but these need not require parental attention.

Sleep difficulties in the young infant are often associated either with excessive nighttime feeding or with unusual habits learned in association with sleep transition (1). Infants are able, by 6 months of age, to sustain adequate nutrition during daytime feedings, so they do not need nighttime feedings. The persistence of nighttime feedings can lead both to expectations on the part of the infant, with habit-associated arousals or difficulty returning to sleep without feeding, and to the arousals associated with excessive voidings and wet diapers due to the feedings. Elimination of the nighttime feedings can solve these problems.

Habits acquired in association with the transition from wakefulness to sleep can be a problem area. Infants who have an elaborate ritual associated with going to sleep may find it difficult to return to sleep following normal awakenings, without a similar ritual. Infants who fall asleep outside of their own bed, e.g., in a room with the lights, radio, or television on, and who are then moved to their crib, may not be able to return to sleep following awakenings without the same conditions being present. Similarly, if the child is always removed from the crib and rocked, cradled, or carried following spontaneous awakening, a habit pattern may be set up in which the infant cannot return to sleep in the absence of these conditions. A careful history will help elucidate such associations, which can then be corrected by the parents. Parents may require considerable support in these efforts, because the infants will typically initially resist the efforts to institute new sleep habits.

A child who has had disturbed sleep in conjunction with a developmental disturbance (e.g., colic—see below), a medical illness, or possibly just a developmental delay in sleep consolidation, may have, in conjunction with the parents, developed atypical habits around sleep onset or awakenings during the night. Such habits can persist, along with the associated sleep disruption, even following resolution of the initial developmental or other problem. Thus, while it may be informative to examine conditions surrounding the onset of a sleep complaint, the persistence of the complaint may be more related to persistence of poor sleep habits rather than to the initial problem itself, which may well have been resolved. Treatment again should be directed toward the poor sleep habits.

Colic in infancy can pose special problems, and because it may affect one in five infants, it deserves mention (2). Colic is characterized by paroxysms of crying, fussing, irritability, increased motor tone, and wakefulness, usually starting in the first several weeks of age, lasting for several months, and usually dissipating by 4 months of age. The etiology is unclear, but a deficiency or developmental delay in CNS inhibitory mechanisms is suspected. Sleep disturbances are common in these infants but should begin to resolve by 4 months of age. If they do not resolve by this time, the parents may be failing to establish a sufficiently regular sleep-wake schedule, based perhaps upon their initial experience with their infant, suggesting that the infant could not adapt to the schedule anyway. This likely would indeed have been true during the first 4 months but may no longer be true. Thus, the parents' experience during the initial 4 months may shape their parenting style in a manner subsequently inappropriate for encouraging normal sleep-wake behavior in their infant.

SLEEP PROBLEMS DURING MIDDLE CHILDHOOD

During the latency period (approximately 4–12 years), sleep is generally good, and few children have complaints. Parasomnias (e.g., night terrors, sleepwalking) are not infrequent during this time period, however, and a careful history of unusual nocturnal behaviors will suggest their presence (see Chapter 5).

Problems that do occur during this period are usually associated with difficulty getting the child to go to sleep, and can often be traced to poor limit setting. A *consistent* bedtime ritual consonant with good sleep hygiene (regular bedtime and arousal time, quiet and darkened sleeping room, no distractions) will help alleviate such problems.

Children are of course also susceptible to having their sleep disturbed by daytime stress factors. Parental interest, concern, and reassurance, as well as allowing the child to talk about difficulties, may be helpful. Occasional transient insomnias—for example, a night on which the child says he or she cannot go to sleep because of worrying about not being able to sleep—can be alleviated by suggesting that instead of thinking about going to sleep, the child should think about a recent pleasurable experience. Sleep will often follow.

The child with severe nighttime fears and unusual fearfulness during the day may present a special problem, and special counseling may be required.

The rare "childhood onset insomnia" may begin during this period (see Chapter 3), but more often than not it will not be complained about by the child, nor may it even be particularly detectable by the parent. These conditions are usually diagnosed retrospectively in adulthood.

SLEEP PROBLEMS DURING ADOLESCENCE

Adolescents are undergoing major developmental changes, experiencing multiple changes in their own roles and in roles expected of them, and entering a time period when other disorders affecting sleep (e.g., narcolepsy) may emerge. Thus stress- and schedule-related insomnia will be more common. Poor sleep hygiene will figure more prominently as an etiological factor. Initial screening of an adolescent with insomnia complaints should emphasize (a) sleep habits and sleep schedule, (b) social and school stress factors, (c) family difficulties, and (d) drug and alcohol use. Disturbances in any area should be carefully evaluated as to their relation to the sleep complaint.

Major mental disorders may emerge during this period, and evidence of disturbed thinking, paranoid ideation, hypomania or grandiosity, or marked difficulties in school should alert the clinician to this possibility. The emergence of schizophrenia may be heralded by frequent terrifying nightmares and a not uncommon associated insomnia. Depression may be seen in adolescent (and even younger) children. However, shortened REM latencies, characteristic of depression in adults, may not characterize depression in children or adolescents.

EDS may be associated with the onset of narcolepsy, which often first presents with falling asleep in school. A not infrequent cause of EDS in adolescents is depression—more so than in adults.

Treatment is appropriately directed first at a primary disorder, if any, underlying the sleep complaint. Stress- and poor sleep hygiene-related insomnias respond well to behavioral techniques, including enforcement of regular schedules, education on good sleep hygiene, sleep restriction, and relaxation or biofeedback training. Counseling may be indicated to resolve family disturbances. Pharmacological agents should probably not be included in the first line of treatment, unless of course they are indicated for an underlying problem such as depression.

CIRCADIAN SCHEDULE DISORDERS IN CHILDREN

Children (infants, latency-age children, and adolescents) are susceptible to circadian sleep disorders such as delayed sleep phase syndrome (3). There is likely a familial component to the tendency to develop these disorders, which, when compounded by family practices that reinforce staying up late and sleeping in the morning, can result in quite profound sleep disturbances. Delayed sleep phase syndrome in adolescents may be associated with a high incidence of depression, which should be kept in mind (4).

Delayed sleep phase syndrome most often begins to cause difficulties when children start school, and when regular early morning awakening becomes important. It is often a struggle to get children to sleep at night, and then equally difficult to awaken them in the morning. They will tend to sleep in on weekends and recoup sleep lost during the week. A careful history and sleep diary will facilitate diagnosis. Family history for similar problems may be positive.

Treatment consists of a regular sleep schedule for both weekdays and weekends, with a regular bedtime and a regular early arising. Chronotherapy of the type used in adults (see Chapter 3) is usually not necessary, but a night of partial sleep restriction, followed by progressively slightly earlier bedtimes, with regularly enforced early morning arising, will often correct the problem over a period of a week or so. Bright-light treatment of circadian sleep disorders in children has not yet been systematically investigated, but it may potentially play a role. The observation that exposure to bright light immediately following completion of the sleep period acts as a phase-advance mechanism suggests that exposure to sunlight in the very early morning might be an appropriate adjunct to other therapy.

Children who are *blind* or *mentally retarded*, or who have *organic CNS disturbances*, can exhibit quite profound circadian schedule disturbances that are frequently manifest as sleep disturbances. Such children may develop free-running non-24-hour sleep-wake rhythms that can be quite disruptive.

ATTENTION DEFICIT DISORDER

Children with attention deficit disorder (ADD) with hyperactivity frequently exhibit disturbed sleep, including difficulty falling asleep, restless sleep, and early morning arising. Children with ADD are frequently treated with stimulant medication, which is also known to alter sleep patterns.

In spite of sleep-related complaints in children with ADD, little polysomnographic evidence exists supporting any particular type of sleep disturbance accompanying the ADD syndrome.

Medications used in the treatment of ADD include stimulants such as methylphenidate (Ritalin) and dextroamphetamine, both known to alter sleep patterns, as well as MAOIs and tricyclics, which are known to suppress REM sleep. Methylphenidate treatment of ADD in children has been shown to delay sleep onset, lengthen sleep, and normalize certain REM sleep parameters. Dextroamphetamine treatment of ADD may result in delayed sleep onset, decreased sleep efficiency, increased REM latency, and decreased REM time. These changes, however, may also be associated with diminished nocturnal arousals and improved overall sleep.

Routine polysomnograms (PSGs) are probably not indicated in ADD, and the stimulant medications used to treat this disorder may not seriously disrupt nocturnal sleep, and might, in fact, tend to decrease nocturnal restlessness. The possibility exists that a subgroup of ADD children may have shorter than normal REM latencies; whether this has therapeutic implications (such as these children being more responsive to tricyclics or MAOIs) remains to be demonstrated.

SLEEP LABORATORY STUDIES IN INFANTS AND CHILDREN

A PSG recording is usually not indicated in most sleep problems in children, especially if a careful clinical evaluation raises a strong suspicion concerning an insomnia possibly related to stress, schedule, or poor sleep hygiene. It is perhaps more reasonable to begin with a good clinical evaluation and then assess clinical response to treatment, reserving polysomnography to cases involving patients who do not respond. Polysomnographic studies are not particularly helpful in sleep complaints associated with mental disorders in this age group.

There are, of course, exceptions. EDS due to narcolepsy or sleep-related breathing disturbances should have a PSG evaluation along with, in the case of narcolepsy, a multiple sleep latency test (MSLT). Restless leg syndrome and associated periodic limb movements of sleep (PLMS; nocturnal myoclonus) can rarely be a cause of insomnia in children. However, one of the present authors (M.R.) had a patient with a severe chronic insomnia, finally diagnosed when the patient was a college senior, as secondary to PLMS. This disorder started with a clear history of a restless leg-type syndrome beginning at the age of 8.

■ ENURESIS

PRESENTING COMPLAINTS

- Wetting the bed at night—evident usually in children
- Frequent urination during the day
- Feelings of guilt or shame by patient

CLINICAL PRESENTATION

The majority of individuals with enuresis have *primary* enuresis, that is, they have never had a consistently dry period. In these patients nighttime bedwetting, expected of an infant or a young child, persists well past the time of normal toilet training. Although there is not strict agreement by clinicians, most feel that enuresis occurring after age 5 deserves evaluation and treatment. These patients often have the need to urinate frequently during the day. Occasional daytime "accidents" are also experienced. The patients may awaken during the night after having wet the bed, or not notice the fact until morning. The enuretic child frequently feels guilty and ashamed about his or her nighttime accidents. As a result the child's social activity may be restricted because he or she will be embarrassed to participate in activities outside the home, such as "sleeping over" at friends' houses, visiting relatives, and camping.

Secondary enuresis is enuresis that has started after the individual has been dry at night for at least 3 months.

INCIDENCE

It is estimated that in the general population 15% of boys and 10% of girls are enuretic at age 5. Approximately 5–10% of enuretic patients have secondary enuresis (5).

ETIOLOGY AND PATHOPHYSIOLOGY

The vast majority of enuretic children have no demonstrable pathology of the urinary tract, especially if there are no symptoms such as urgency, abnormalities in stream or flow, or daytime enuresis. Most enuretic children have a small *functional* bladder capacity, which may be considered as a maturational delay of bladder development. Some studies have suggested that enuretic children have more and stronger bladder contractions than nonenuretic children. The bladder of the enuretic child can be thought of as one that fills quickly, contracts vigorously, and faces little resistance.

Secondary enuresis raises the index of suspicion that an organic problem may be involved or that the enuresis is in response to a stress or a conflict situation.

Anatomic conditions that uncommonly are associated with enuresis include a congenitally small bladder, wide bladder neck anomalies, bladder outflow obstruction, urethral diverticula, ectopic ureters, and epispadias. Medical conditions such as urinary tract infections, diabetes mellitus, and diabetes insipidus also are associated with enuresis. Obstructive sleep apnea occasionally has enuresis as a coexistent symptom.

SLEEP LABORATORY FINDINGS

Laboratory studies have demonstrated that the sleep of enuretic children is normal. Because enuresis occurs in all stages of sleep, sleep laboratory studies are not thought to be indicated in most enuretic children.

DIFFERENTIAL DIAGNOSIS

The history of continuing enuresis with no intervening dry periods, especially with positive family history, strongly suggests primary enuresis. Abnormalities of flow and/or urgency, or presence of other symptoms, raise the index of suspicion of other medical etiologies.

Nocturnal seizures with urinary incontinence should be differentiated from simple enuresis. Patients with nocturnal epilepsy often will have a history of diurnal seizures as well. There may be evidence of vigorous motor activity or tongue biting during sleep. A clinical daytime EEG or expanded PSG is occasionally needed to determine if nocturnal seizures are the cause of the enuresis.

TREATMENT

Most clinicians use a standard plan in the treatment of enuresis. A flow chart for the treatment of enuresis is illustrated in Figure 8-1.

Step 1: Initial evaluation. This should include a thorough medical and sleep history (especially with respect to symptoms of diabetes mellitus, seizures, snoring, or urinary tract infection) and a complete physical exam. A 2-week data log used to record times of meals (snacks included), number of bathroom trips (both daytime and nighttime), hours of sleep, and whether bedwetting occurred, should be obtained and reviewed. A urine sample should be evaluated for glucosuria or signs of infection. A quantitative measurement of the urine volume should be made to estimate the functional bladder capacity. This can be done at home by parent or child by measuring the amount of urine voided in a measuring cup. The rule of thumb is that children 6–12 years old have a bladder capacity about 1 ounce per year of age. If abnormalities are found upon physical examination or urinalysis, further evaluation or specialty consultation should be obtained.

Step 2: Discussion of the nature of enuresis and the treatment plan with the patient and his or her parents. A system of rewards to be given to the child for dry nights should be agreed upon. The child's participation should be encouraged by asking the child to

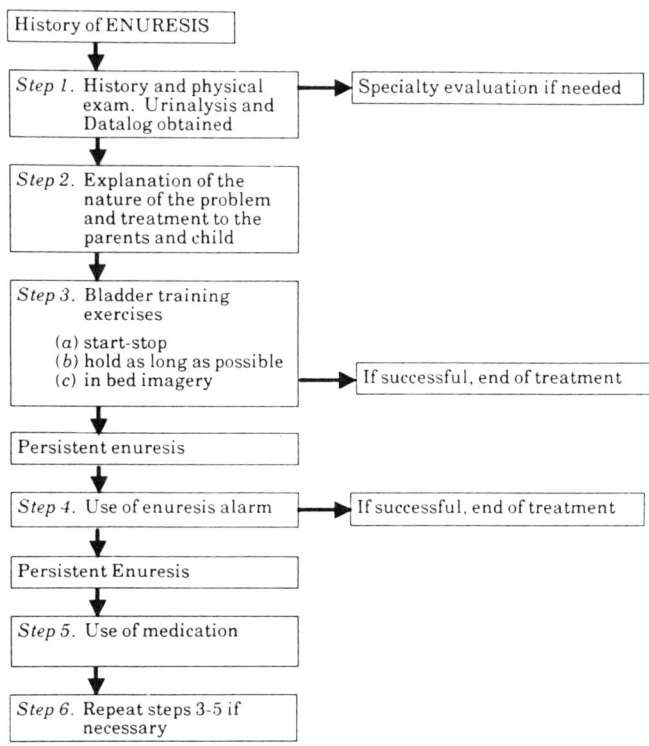

FIGURE 8-1. **Flowchart for the treatment of enuresis.**

state why he or she wants to overcome the enuresis. Often asking the child to change his or her bed clothes or bedding relieves the guilt that the child feels of having a parent clean up after him or her.

Step 3: Bladder training exercises. The child is asked to do a "start and stop" exercise (5–10 times per micturition) every time he or she urinates. This exercise may strengthen the external sphincter and give the child the sensation of controlling micturition. Twice a week the child is given a large amount of his or her favorite liquid to drink. The child is then asked to retain the urine as long as possible before voiding. Weekly measurements of the amount voided should be recorded to observe if the functional bladder capacity is increasing. Another exercise is to have the child lie in bed after he or she has consumed a large quantity of liquid. The child pretends to be asleep and practices holding his or her urine until he or she gets up and goes to the bathroom. Often with these bladder training exercises alone, the functional bladder capacity will increase, the number of bathroom trips during the day will decrease, and the enuresis will cease.

Step 4: Enuresis alarm. If after a few weeks of bladder training exercises the child is still having wet nights, an enuresis alarm can be used. The most effective alarms are those that are triggered by a small amount of urine, with the sensor located in the underclothes. The alarm should be positioned close to the ear (usually clipped to the shirt collar). The child must get up and go to the bathroom when he or she is awakened by the alarm. The combination of the bladder training exercises and an enuresis alarm is very effective in treating primary enuresis.

Step 5: Medication. This option can be considered in the rare cases when enuresis persists after bladder exercises and alarms have been utilized. Imipramine has been commonly used in the past (25–50 mg 30 minutes prior to bed), although its mechanism of action is not known. Oxybutynin chloride has been used in patients refractory to imipramine.

Step 6: If after initial success the child has a relapse, the earlier steps should be repeated.

■ SLEEP IN THE ELDERLY

PRESENTING COMPLAINTS

Elderly patients exhibit an increase in sleep complaints as well as both objectively poorer sleep and increases in medical and other problems known to adversely affect sleep. Presenting complaints often include the following:

- Difficulty falling asleep and staying asleep

- Early morning awakening with difficulty returning to sleep
- Unrefreshing sleep
- Excessive tiredness or fatigue during the day
- Unusual behaviors occurring during the sleep period
- Unusual nocturnal behaviors

CLINICAL PRESENTATION

Most of the sleep problems seen in younger adults may affect the elderly, as well as special problems unique to or of much greater frequency in the elderly. Proper clinical evaluation is very important in elderly patients. It is especially important not to pass off sleep complaints as a "normal" part of aging, or to merely prescribe a hypnotic medication without first properly evaluating the complaint, because correctable underlying disorders may be missed and/or aggravated.

Elderly patients may complain directly about their sleep problems. However, some need to be questioned directly about these problems, because they may consider them a "normal" part of getting older, and thus not worth bringing up. Frequently, family members (when the elderly are living at home) or nursing staff (when the elderly are in hospitals or nursing homes) will be the ones to complain about unusual sleep habits or behaviors. It is important to listen carefully to such complaints, because important cues as to etiology may be found in the complaint.

INCIDENCE

The incidence of insomnia complaints increases dramatically in the elderly. The number of older individuals with insomnia complaints, as obtained from surveys, has ranged from 25% of those over 70 in a Florida study (6) to 48% of those over 50 in a Los Angeles study (7).

Several, but not all, studies have found substantial increases in both sleep apnea and PLMS (nocturnal myoclonus) in asymptomatic, otherwise healthy elderly individuals. The range of increase varies considerably, however, up to 20–30% or more of the elderly population. It is not yet clear that this increase in these disorders is a normal part of the aging process (8, 9, 10).

ETIOLOGY AND PATHOPHYSIOLOGY

The etiology of sleep complaints in the elderly can be attributed to four main mechanisms:

1. The aging process may be associated with normal alterations in physiological systems controlling sleep and sleep behaviors.
2. Specific sleep disorders, such as nocturnal myoclonus and sleep apnea, appear to have an increased incidence in the elderly.
3. Psychiatric and medical disorders that adversely influence sleep have an increased incidence in the elderly.
4. The elderly are frequently on a variety of medications, for a variety of reasons, that may either interact or act differently in the elderly person, resulting in altered sleep patterns or sleep behavior.

Sleep EEG morphology changes with age: Stage 3 and Stage 4 sleep diminishes in amount, and stages of lighter sleep increase in proportion. Wakefulness and number of arousals, as well as sleep fragmentation, increase with age. These changes may be associated with a perceived lessened quality and/or quantity of sleep. Increased arousals and consequent sleep fragmentation result in an increased level of daytime sleepiness. There may be a tendency for decreased REM latency in elderly individuals, but this decrease is usually not in the range seen with major affective disorder.

The neurobiological systems that control the timing of circadian biorhythms, including the sleep-wake cycle, may become less efficient with age and less able to adapt to change. There is evidence of a dampened circadian rest-activity rhythm with advancing age, and of a similar dampening of the circadian body temperature rhythm, with higher nocturnal body temperature. Thus elderly individuals may be more susceptible to interruptions in their circadian schedules. This possibly increased susceptibility is especially important in patients in nursing homes, where clear day-night differences in light, noise, and activity may be diminished by the environment. There is also evidence of decreases in the secretion of growth hormone associated with slow wave sleep in the elderly, as well as a possible increase in resting plasma norepinephrine, a marker of central sympathetic activity. This latter finding could be related to both the sleep fragmentation and the increased nighttime body temperature seen in the elderly (11).

The increase in PLMS and restless leg syndrome seen with age may impact sleep quality, usually resulting in what is perceived as insomnia. The increased frequency of sleep apnea is not necessarily associated with evidence of hemodynamic or cardiovascular consequences, although it may be associated with increased daytime sleepiness.

Psychiatric disorders, especially depression, are more frequent in the elderly, along with the sleep disturbances associated with these disorders, such as early morning awakening. Medical disorders, especially those associated with chronic pain (e.g., osteoarthritis), are more frequent in the elderly, again interfering with sleep. Nocturia may aggravate an otherwise unapparent problem in falling back to sleep. Skin disorders associated with itching may aggravate sleep. The extent to which such medically related symptoms can be controlled will be beneficial to sleep, but often the very medications used for control of medical symptoms will aggravate sleep further.

It is very important to consider the role of medications in inducing sleep problems in the elderly. It has been estimated that 10% of the elderly population in the United States consume a quarter of the prescription drugs prescribed. Prescription and nonprescription drugs that are frequently used by the elderly and that may induce sleep problems are listed in Table 8-1.

TABLE 8-1. **Prescription and nonprescription drugs that may induce sleep problems in the elderly**

Caffeine	Nicotine
Alcohol	Scopolamine agents
Some antihypertensives	Steroids
Stimulants	Xanthine derivatives
Thyroid hormone	Methysergide
Antiarrhythmic agents	Nasal decongestants

While hypnotic use is increased in the elderly, the ability to metabolize hypnotics may diminish, especially in the presence of renal or hepatic disease. Thus a single dose may act longer and have greater effect. The possibility of drug interactions (e.g., competition for hepatic microsomal enzyme systems in impaired hepatic function) increases in the elderly.

LABORATORY FINDINGS

Polysomnographic studies of nocturnal sleep in healthy elderly individuals have shown decreases in sleep efficiency, increases in number of awakenings and total time awake (especially in the last 2 hours of the night), and marked diminution in Stage 3 and Stage 4 sleep. These changes, which usually begin somewhere around 50 years of age, are age-related and are generally more pronounced in men.

The role of the sleep laboratory in evaluating sleep complaints in the elderly is similar to the role it plays in general. The use of a sleep laboratory should be considered if there is a high degree of suspicion that specific abnormalities exist, such as apnea or myoclonus, that require a PSG for documentation. First, however, other possible causes of the complaint must be assessed. Medical conditions and treatment efficacy must be evaluated, medications may need to be changed or reduced, and sleep hygiene and sleep schedules should be improved before considering a PSG.

Polysomnographic interpretation in the elderly is complicated by both the sleep-disrupting effects of concurrent illness and the medications used in treatment of this age group.

If a PSG is obtained, shortened REM latency may be helpful in suggesting an affective disorder component to a sleep complaint. It may also be helpful in separating early dementia (normal REM latency) from depression (shortened REM latency).

DIFFERENTIAL DIAGNOSIS

The differential diagnosis of sleep complaints in the elderly is among the most demanding of tasks in sleep disorders medicine, to the extent that rigor, thoroughness, and a high index of suspicion are necessary.

A decision tree similar to that proposed for the differential diagnosis of chronic insomnia (see Figure 3-1) is appropriate, paying special attention to the following issues, which must be systematically explored:

- Have poor sleep habits contributed to the complaint? Spending excessive time in bed, keeping the radio or television on, excessive daytime napping, and lack of exercise are examples.
- Have coexisting medical disorders been adequately evaluated and optimally treated? Might some be unrecognized? Can treatment of these disorders be interfering with sleep?
- To what extent are medications (prescription or otherwise), sedative-hypnotics, alcohol, and/or nicotine contributing to the complaint? A trial reduction or elimination of all but clearly medically necessary drugs is often helpful in differential diagnosis.
- Is unrecognized depression or dementia playing a role?

TREATMENT

Treatment generally resembles that of similar sleep disorders in other patients, with special attention to several specific areas. Often treatment includes substantial modification of sleep hygiene/sleep environment, which may be resisted and may need considerable explanation, and for which the patient may need reassurance. Treatment of the sleep complaint apart from other medical disorders and complaints is difficult; considerable interchange with other physicians may be necessary. Those patients seeing several different specialists and receiving one or more prescriptions from each pose special problems—ideally (rarely the case), one physician should manage all medications. The role of pharmacological agents must be tempered by the fact that half-lives may be extended, the possibility of multiple drug interactions is increased, and lower than accustomed doses may be adequate.

Therapeutic intervention for relatively mild apnea in the

elderly, considering the infrequent association with significant physiological consequences, must be carefully considered on an individual basis (12).

■ SLEEP PROBLEMS DURING PREGNANCY

PRESENTING COMPLAINTS

- Excessive sleepiness early in pregnancy
- Difficulty falling asleep or staying sleep, usually beginning in the second or third trimester
- Backaches and/or physical discomfort interfering with sleep

CLINICAL PRESENTATION

The first few weeks of pregnancy are often accompanied by complaints of excessive tiredness and increased need for sleep. Often these symptoms accompany those of nausea and morning sickness of early pregnancy. By the third trimester, sleep complaints are probably the rule, but by now the primary complaint tends to be insomnia or difficulty sleeping, difficulty falling asleep or frequent awakening, or both. Sleep complaints secondary to nonpregnancy-related causes of disturbed sleep or insomnia may complicate the picture as well. Thus one's index of suspicion for other disorders should be high.

INCIDENCE

Up to two-thirds of pregnant women consider their sleep to be abnormal. Complaints include physical discomfort and backaches, awakenings typically described as "just waking up," urinary frequency, awakenings from fetal movements, heartburn, cramps or tingling in the legs, and difficulty getting to sleep (13). It appears that about 75% of these complaints can be related to the anatomical and physiological changes associated with pregnancy, but about 25% of the complaints are seemingly unrelated to the size of the uterus. By the third trimester, sleep complaints are the rule rather than the exception.

ETIOLOGY AND PATHOPHYSIOLOGY

The hormone progesterone may be related to the excessive sleepiness of early pregnancy; a metabolite of progesterone has been found to act as a barbiturate-like ligand of the GABA receptor in the brain (14). Usually the excessive sleepiness resolves spontaneously.

As mentioned above, most sleep complaints later in pregnancy (especially in the third trimester) stem from the anatomical and physiological changes induced by the growing baby. It is clear that as pregnancy progresses it becomes more and more difficult to find a comfortable sleep posture. The weight of the fetus and the enlarged uterus pressing on surrounding structures becomes uncomfortable. It is no longer possible to sleep on the stomach, and sleeping on the back and side becomes uncomfortable. As the baby's head begins to press on the bladder, more frequent trips to the bathroom become likely.

Not infrequently, a type of primary insomnia of pregnancy may be seen as well, but the pathophysiology of this insomnia is not yet understood.

There is, of course, nothing to prevent a pregnant woman from having other causes of disordered sleep, such as an affective disorder, a circadian rhythm-based disorder, or nocturnal myoclonus, and the clinician must keep this possibility in mind. Additionally, problems are sometimes encountered in patients who are being treated with hypnotics or tricyclics who then become pregnant, with recommendations that the medications be discontinued.

LABORATORY FINDINGS

Polysomnographic studies of sleep during pregnancy are quite limited. There is evidence of decreases in Stage 4 sleep in late pregnancy, as well as more time awake and more frequent awakenings.

It is rare that diagnostic polysomnography would be required during pregnancy. If such is the case, then it primarily is needed for differential diagnosis of other suspected medical causes for the sleep complaint (e.g., narcolepsy, nocturnal myoclonus, sleep-related breathing disorder). In such cases standard diagnostic criteria would generally apply.

DIFFERENTIAL DIAGNOSIS

Accurate differential diagnosis of pregnancy-related sleep complaints begins with an appreciation of what the "normal" sleep complaints during pregnancy are, and whether or not the patient's complaints differ from the normal ones. A detailed sleep history is important. Did the symptoms arise within the pregnancy, or did they antedate or become aggravated by the pregnancy? Is there reason to believe that the patient may be suffering from a concurrent sleep disorder unrelated to the pregnancy? It is important to ask about early morning awakenings (affective disorder), duration of complaint (does it antedate pregnancy?), and possible association with stress or loss. One will want to be aware of acute or gradual onset, and whether the problem improves when the patient is away from home or the normal sleep environment (psychophysiological insomnia). Snoring, breathing pauses, excessive movement, shortness of breath or palpitations upon awakening, and morning headaches may be suggestive of disorders that would be best diagnosed by use of a nocturnal PSG. Evidence of chronic anxiety, panic attacks, or depression, including vegetative signs, would lead to thoughts of an anxiety or depressive disorder, which may suggest a psychiatric consultation.

Special pregnancy-related anxieties may relate to the feeling of being out of control of one's own physiology. The pregnant woman finds herself losing her customary figure, susceptible to increased mood changes, at times plagued by nausea and vomiting, unable to sleep, as well as being discouraged from using customary medications that may help her sleep. She may also have concerns about being a good mother, and fears about how her husband will react to the baby. She may be afforded no comfort from well-meaning friends who nonetheless regale her with horror stories of how their children did not sleep through the night until they were 2 years old.

TREATMENT

The treatment of sleep complaints during pregnancy is complicated by the fact that most pharmacological agents should be used with great care and caution. The use of sleep hygiene and other behavioral techniques should be emphasized whenever possible. It is, of course, essential to recognize when a sleep complaint may be symptomatic of a more serious underlying disorder, such as a major affective disorder. In these cases, more vigorous intervention is mandatory, including pharmacological intervention if appropriate.

The most important aspect of treatment is, again, proper assessment and accurate diagnosis. If the sleep complaints fall within the "normal" range, education and reassurance that things will improve after delivery will be helpful. Seeing a light at the end of the tunnel can be most encouraging. The sleep position problems during the third trimester can often be best handled by judicious use of extra pillows. Evening fluid intake can be decreased. Customary sleep hygiene techniques should be emphasized (see Chapter 3).

There is a *special role for the father* in the management of sleep disorders in pregnancy. The husband can help his pregnant wife with insomnia by providing support, by being available to her, and by helping her reduce some of the pressures resulting from her impaired daytime functioning. The father may feel alienated by his wife's preoccupation with the unborn child and her impending relationship with the new child. It is important that the husband not view his wife's insomnia-related fatigue as additional rejection or as evidence of emotional distancing. Appropriate counseling by the perceptive physician may be helpful in this regard.

If the sleep disorder is the result of a psychiatric disturbance or a primary sleep disorder requiring medication, it is important that the husband be involved in making the decisions with respect to medication use. Potential hazards should be explained, and both husband and wife should be made to understand that medication is frequently a last resort.

At times the pregnant woman may complain that her sleep is disturbed by her *husband's disruptive sleep patterns* or snoring.

In such cases, appropriate evaluation of the husband's sleep may be in order.

Sleep problems seemingly independent of or in addition to those associated with pregnancy per se require special attention. Sleep restriction, relaxation, and perhaps even biofeedback may be appropriate for cases in which a significant psychophysiological insomnia component is likely present.

PHARMACOLOGICAL AGENTS

Medications pose special problems. Benzodiazepine use during the first trimester has been found to be correlated with an increased incidence of oral clefts, and is probably contraindicated. There is no good evidence of problems associated with the use of benzodiazepines during the second trimester, but one should still prescribe with caution during this period. During the third trimester, benzodiazepine use has been associated with abstinence syndromes in the newborn, as well as transient neurological signs. This association would suggest that benzodiazepine use be terminated as early as possible in the third trimester (15).

Tricyclics are frequently used in depressed patients with insomnia. Developmental abnormalities do not appear to be associated with imipramine or amitriptyline use during the first trimester, although there is evidence of tricyclic withdrawal syndrome in infants whose mothers had used tricyclics during the third trimester. Discontinuing use of tricyclics at least 10 days before anticipated delivery would appear to be warranted.

Alcohol use may be associated with the fetal alcohol syndrome, and even small amounts of alcohol may be associated with increases in teratogenicity. The use of alcohol appears contraindicated.

There is insufficient evidence to state with certainty that any sedative-hypnotic agent is absolutely free of any teratogenic effect; thus the use of this type of agent should be discouraged. The role of tryptophan in pregnancy has not been well documented. Because tryptophan is present in the normal diet in amounts up to ½ to 2 g per day, an additional 1 to 2 g would seem unlikely to be harmful, and it might be considered worthy of trial in patients responding poorly to nonpharmacological intervention.

SLEEP AFTER DELIVERY

Patients can be reassured that their sleep will likely improve rapidly after delivery, and this is usually the case, assuming other causes of a sleep disorder are not present. This fact alone will often be of substantial benefit to the patient with a pregnancy-related sleep complaint. However, the presence of the new baby likely will be another source of disturbed sleep, until such time as the infant learns it is appropriate to sleep at night and be active during the day. It is helpful to tell the mother what to expect in this regard.

■ INSOMNIA WITHOUT OBJECTIVE FINDINGS

There is a group of patients who have a chronic insomnia complaint, but who have no objective evidence of sleep abnormality on the PSG. This syndrome was formerly termed "pseudoinsomnia," and reference to this term may still be found. The incidence is not well established, as patients with this syndrome typically respond well to behavioral treatments for psychophysiological insomnia. Thus, if an insomnia complaint is managed according to the decision tree we have outlined earlier in Chapter 3, with PSGs being reserved primarily for those patients who do not respond to treatment for psychophysiological insomnia (unless a PSG is otherwise indicated), such patients will not be identified. When large groups of patients with insomnia complaints are studied polysomnographically, however, before treatment, the incidence can be as high as 19% of patients recorded (16). The PSG in such cases indicates essentially normal sleep, with the patient insisting that sleep on the night in question was either too short, or otherwise of poor quality.

These patients may represent individuals who have difficulty in distinguishing the sleep state from wakefulness, or individuals in whom short arousals interspersed between longer sleep periods are associated with a subjective continuity of consciousness, and lack of awareness of the intervening (and much longer) sleep periods. Some investigators have suggested that some yet undetected abnormality of sleep occurs in these individuals.

The complaint of insomnia should be taken seriously in these patients, even if polysomnographic findings are absent or equivocal. While occasionally the information that sleep, as characterized on the PSG, was found to be normal is helpful to such patients, more typically a course of treatment as outlined for psychophysiological insomnia is indicated.

■ REFERENCES

1. Ferber R: The sleepless child, in Sleep and its Disorders in Children. Edited by Guilleminault C. New York, Raven Press, 1987, pp 141–163
2. Weissbluth M: Sleep and the colicky infant, in Sleep and its Disorders in Children. Edited by Guilleminault C. New York, Raven Press, 1987, pp 129–140
3. Ferber R: Circadian and schedule disturbances, in Sleep and its Disorders in Children. Edited by Guilleminault C. New York, Raven Press, 1987, pp 165–175
4. Thorpy MJ, Korman E, Spielman AJ, et al: Delayed sleep phase syndrome in adolescents. J Adolesc Health Care 9:22–27, 1988
5. Nino-Murcia G, Keenan S: Enuresis and sleep, in Sleep and its Disorders in Children. Edited by Guilleminault C. New York, Raven Press, 1987, pp 253–267
6. Karacan I, Thornby JI, Anch M, et al: Prevalence of sleep disturbances in a primarily urban Florida county. Soc Sci Med 10:239–244, 1976
7. Bixler EO, Kales A, Soldatos CR, et al: Prevalence of sleep disorders in the Los Angeles metropolitan area. Am J Psychiatry 136:1257–1262, 1979
8. Ancoli-Israel S, Kripke DF, Mason W: Characteristics of obstructive and central sleep apnea in the elderly: an interim report. Biol Psychiatry 22:741–750, 1987
9. Reynolds CF, Kupfer DJ, Taska LS, et al: Sleep of healthy seniors: a revisit. Sleep 8:20–29, 1985
10. Mosko SS, Dickel MJ, Ashorst J: Night to night variability in sleep apnea and sleep-related periodic leg movements in the elderly. Sleep 11:340–348, 1988
11. Vitiello MV, Prinz PN: Aging and sleep disorders, in Sleep Disorders: Diagnosis and Treatment, 2nd Edition. Edited by Williams H, Karacan I. New York, John Wiley, 1988, pp 293–312
12. Knight H, Millman RP, Gur RC, et al: Clinical significance of sleep apnea in the elderly. Am Rev Respir Dis 136:845–850, 1987

13. Schweiger MS: Sleep disturbances in pregnancy. Am J Obstet Gynecol 114:879–882, 1972
14. Majewska MD, Harrison NL, Schwartz RD, et al: Steroid hormone metabolites are barbiturate-like modulators of the GABA receptor. Science 232:1004–1007, 1986
15. Calabrese JC, Gulledge AD: Psychotropics during pregnancy and lactation. A review. Psychosomatics 26:413–426, 1985
16. Zorick F, Kribbs N, Roehrs T, et al: Polysomnographic and MMPI characteristics of patients with insomnia. Psychopharmacology (Berlin) (suppl) 1:2–10, 1984

INDEX

Abnormal swallowing, 119–120
Adolescents
  circadian disorders in, 157
  depression in, 11, 40, 96, 141, 156–157
  EDS in, 77, 96, 156
  sleep problems of, 156
  sleep stages of, 20
  sleepwalking, 113
Advanced sleep phase syndrome, 44–45
Alcohol avoidance, 68, 87, 173
Alcohol-induced sleep disorders, 3, 31, 33–35
Alpha-delta sleep, 36, 124
Alpha rhythm, 14
American Sleep Disorders Association (ASDA), 3, 6, 8
Anorexia nervosa, 125
Apnea
  a cause of EDS, 101
  central apnea, 6, 32, 59–62, 89, 93, 99–100
  diagnosis, 11, 96–97
  incidence of, 93
  laboratory findings, 93–96
  mixed apnea, 93, 95
  obstructive apnea, 5, 89–91, 93–95, 99–100
  paraphysiology and etiology, 91–93
  snoring a symptom of, 32, 90, 93, 102
  treatment, 97–100
Arousal disorders, 4, 113. *See also* Night terrors; Sleepwalking
Arthritis, 125
Ascending reticular activating system (ARAS), 20–21
Asthma, 93, 96, 123
Attention deficit disorder (ADD), 158
Atypical depression, 140–141
Automatic behavior, 82, 115

Benzodiazepine agents, 28, 33, 35–39, 144–146, 173
Biofeedback, 58, 69–70, 156, 173
Bipolar disorder, 133
Breathing disorders, 11, 89–100. *See also* Apnea; Hypersomnia

Bright light therapy, 43–45, 49
Bronchospasm, 100
Bruxism, 119

Caffeine, 49, 68, 104
Carbon dioxide, 9, 93
Cardiac-related symptoms, 9, 93, 96, 110–111
  See also Tachycardia
Cataplexy, 81–82, 88–89
Central nervous system (CNS)
  arousal of the, 24
  depressants, 46, 97, 105
  disturbances, 157
  hypersomnia, 97, 101–102
  inhibitory mechanisms, 154
  neoplasms, 123
  serotonergic, 102
  sleep systems based in the, 5
  stimulants, 46
Children
  apnea in, 99
  bruxism in, 119
  EDS in, 78
  enuretic, 159–163
  insomnia in, 73
  REM latency in, 20, 156, 158
  sleep problems of, 3, 77, 152–159
  sleepwalking, 112–113
Chronotherapy, 43
Cigarettes, 47, 69
Circadian disorders
  among the dyssomnias, 3
  in children, 157
  in the elderly, 165
  physiology of, 22–24
  presented as insomnias, 2
  types of, 40–50
  See also Delayed sleep phase syndrome
Clitoral erections, 22
Continuous positive airway pressure (CPAP), 99
Contraceptive agents, 104
Cyclothymia, 134
Cystic fibrosis, 123

Daytime sleepiness. *See* Excessive daytime sleepiness; Hypersomnia
Death, 21–22, 120
Delayed sleep phase syndrome, 3, 31, 40–44
Delta sleep, 16, 20
Dementia, 109, 167–168
Depression
  in adolescents, 11, 40, 96, 156–157
  associated with hypersomnolence, 97
  atypical, 140–141
  in children, 157
  diagnosis, 12
  EDS secondary to, 96
  in the elderly, 166–167
  masked, 134
  related to insomnia, 30, 127–129, 131–133
  in SADs, 139–140
  See also REM latency
Diabetes, 123, 161
Diagnosis and management, 1, 4–6, 28–29
Diagnostic nomenclature, 2–4
Dreaming, 24–25
Drug dependency. *See* Substance abuse
Drug history, 31
Drug screen, 10
Drug use in treatment, 38–39, 142–152
Dyssomnias, 3
Dysthymia, 127, 134

Epstein-Barr virus (EBV), 124
Elderly persons, 151, 163–169
Endocrinopathies, 123
Endogenous disorders, 3
Enuresis, 4, 90, 159–163
Epileptic seizures, 115
Excessive daytime sleepiness (EDS)
  in adolescents, 156
  complaints of, 1, 76
  due to narcolepsy, 156, 159
  in the elderly, 165
  evaluation of, 76–79
  and hypoventilation, 91

Excessive daytime sleepiness (EDS) *(continued)*
  psychiatric disorders associated with, 139–141
  as a symptom, 5
  testing of, 10–11
  See also Apnea; Hypersomnia; Narcolepsy
Exogenous disorders, 3

Fibrositis, 123–124

Gastric acid, 125

Hallucinations, 81–83, 96, 119
Headache, 90, 125
Hormones, 24–26
Hyperactivity, 34, 158
Hypersomnia, 84, 89–106, 109, 133, 141. *See also* Apnea; Central nervous system; Excessive daytime sleepiness
Hyperventilation, 129
Hypnotics. *See* Sedative-hypnotic agents; Substance abuse
Hypomania, 134, 139–140
Hypopnea, 95
Hypoventilation, 91
Hypoxemia, 91, 93, 96, 100

Immunological function, 25
Infants, 19–20, 120, 152–155, 157–158
Insomnia
  childhood onset, 73, 155
  chronic, 1, 28–33, 36, 41, 143
  drug-related, 34–40
  high altitude, 3, 28
  pain-induced, 29, 122, 166
  psychiatric disorders associated with, 30, 127–139
  psychophysiological, 3, 11, 32–33, 62–72
  rare causes of, 72
  rebound, 35, 37–39, 146
  REM interruption, 73–74
  sleep onset, 40, 52, 144
  stress-related, 28
  transient, 27–28, 143
  See also Apnea

Insufficient sleep. *See* Sleep deprivation
Irregular sleep-wake cycle, 46

Jet lag, 3, 23, 40, 49–50

Kleine-Levin syndrome, 103–104

Mean sleep latency (MSL), 10
Medical disorders, 4, 29, 122–127
Melatonin, 24
Menstruation, 104
Microsleeps, 26, 76, 81. *See also* Naps
Minnesota Multiphasic Personality Inventory (MMPI), 64, 66, 114, 127
Multiple sleep latency test (MSLT), 6, 10–11, 78–79, 159
Myoclonus. *See* Periodic limb movements of sleep

Naps
   in diagnosis of apnea, 96
   in narcolepsy and its treatment, 81, 87–88
   as part of the MSLT, 10
   for shift workers, 49
   in sleep history, 77
   See also Microsleeps
Narcolepsy
   an endogenous disorder, 3
   complaints and clinical presentation, 80–82
   diagnosis, 11, 84–86
   etiology and pathophysiology, 83–84
   incidence, 83
   laboratory findings, 84
   related to REM sleep, 5, 81, 83–86
   treatment, 86–89
Neonatal sleep myoclonus, 120
Neoplasms, 123
Neurophysiology, 20–27
Nightmares
   associated with psychiatric disorders, 127
   associated with REM sleep, 19, 25, 35, 108, 148
   diagnosis, 115

as parasomnia, 108
Night terrors, 25, 111–117, 120
Nocturnal death, 120
Nocturnal myoclonus. *See* Periodic limb movements of sleep
Non-24-hour sleep-wake cycle, 40, 45

Oxygen desaturation, 92–93
Oxygen saturation, 9, 92, 96

Panic attacks, 115, 135–137
Parasomnias, 2, 4, 11, 18, 108–122
Parkinson's disease, 123
Paroxysmal dystonia, 120
Penile erection, 8, 10, 22, 110
Peptide substances, 25
Periodic limb movements of sleep (PLMS)
   an endogenous disorder, 3
   cause of EDS, 105–106
   cause of insomnia, 3, 31–33, 51–58
   diagnosis, 11–12
   in the elderly, 166
   rare in children, 159
   See also Restless leg syndrome
Physiology and pathology, 14–27
Polysomnography (PSG)
   in breathing disorders, 11, 96
   a diagnostic aid, 6
   in drug dependency insomnia, 36
   in EDS complaints, 78–79
   in PLMS disorders, 31–32, 54
   rarely used for parasomnias, 11
   REM latency seen by, 84
Posttraumatic stress disorder, 138
Pregnancy, 169–174
Prolactin, 24–25
Psychiatric disorders, 4, 30, 127–141, 166
Psychiatric evaluation, 128
Psychiatric referral, 1, 171
Psychological tests, 64
Pulmonary disorders, 93–96, 123

Rapid eye movement (REM)
  during dreaming, 24
  interruption, 32, 73–74
  parasomnias associated with, 4, 108–111
  periods, 11–12, 18
  rebound, 34–38, 68, 105, 148
  related to sleep functions, 25–26
  related to sleep stages, 10, 14–22
  sleep behavior disorder, 109, 116
  sleep related to narcolepsy, 5, 81, 83–86
  suppression, 68, 142, 144
REM latency
  in children, 20
  in the elderly, 165
  length of, 12, 36, 158
  not seen on the PSG, 84
  related to depression, 25, 132–134, 156, 167
  related to schizophrenia, 131
Renal failure, 125
Restless leg syndrome, 31, 51–58, 159. *See also* Periodic limb movements of sleep
Rhythm-based disorders. *See* Circadian disorders
Rhythmic movement disorder, 118

Saliva, 119
Schizophrenia, 103, 130–131, 156
Seasonal affective disorders (SADs), 139–140
Sedative-hypnotic agents
  insomnia caused by, 5, 35–36
  sleep disorders caused by, 31, 33–34
  use of, 142–152
  withdrawal from, 39
  See also Substance abuse
Shift work, 3, 40, 46–49, 66
Sinus arrest, 92, 110
Sleep architecture, 14–20, 95
Sleep cycles, 18–19. *See also* Sleep-wake cycles
Sleep deprivation, 10, 26, 31, 101
Sleep diary, 7, 29
Sleep Disorders Centers, 2, 8–12, 33
Sleep drunkenness, 82, 102, 115
Sleep events. *See* Parasomnias

Sleep functions, 25–26
Sleep history, 6–7, 29, 128, 161
Sleep hygiene
  in circadian desynchronization, 42–43
  as part of sleep history, 7
  principles of, 67–69
  related to sleep disorders, 3, 28, 78, 155–156
Sleepiness disorders, 76–107, 127. *See also* Excessive daytime sleepiness
Sleep limits, 3. *See also* Sleep restriction
Sleep onset insomnia, 40, 52, 144
Sleep paralysis
  an hallucination, 119
  in narcoleptics, 81–83, 102, 109
  a parasomnia, 4
  presentation of, 108–109
  related to apnea, 96
  treatment, 88, 109
Sleep patterns, 19–20
Sleep physiology, 21–24
Sleep restriction, 70–71, 156. *See also* Sleep limits
Sleep stages, 3, 12, 14–22
Sleep starts, 118
Sleep talking, 4, 111, 118
Sleep-wake cycles, 45–46. *See also* Sleep cycles
Sleep-wake rhythm, 22, 153
Sleep-wake schedule, 2, 47
Sleep-wake transition, 4
Sleepwalking, 111–118
Snoring
  absent in EDS, 91
  as a parasomnia, 4, 121
  as a symptom of apnea, 32, 90, 93, 102
  as a symptom of enuresis, 161
Somnolence, 101–102
Substance abuse, 3, 10–11, 33–40, 104–105. *See also* Sedative-hypnotic agents
Symptom approach to disorders, 2–6

Tachycardia, 30, 92, 112, 125, 137. *See also* Cardiac-related symptoms
Testosterone, 25
Tonic spasms, 120
Tracheostomy, 99

Violent behavior, 112
Viral infections, 25, 102

Wakefulness, 14, 20, 26, 32, 52